A Future Agenda

Report of the
Commission on

Education
For Health
Administration
Volume I, 1975

Selected Papers of the
Commission on

Education
For Health
Administration
Volume II, 1975

Published for, and with the support of, the
W. K. Kellogg Foundation

Health Administration Press
M2240-School of Public Health
The University of Michigan
Ann Arbor, MI 48109
1977

Education
For Health
Administration
Volume III

A
Future
Agenda

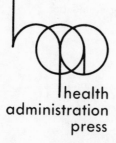

health
administration
press

School of Public Health
The University of Michigan
1977

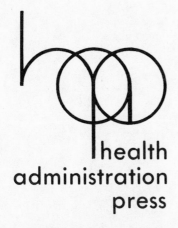

Contents

Foreword

In June of 1976, two years after the Commission on Education for Health Administration reported its findings and recommendations, the W. K. Kellogg Foundation sponsored the North American Invitational Conference on Health Administration Education at Oak Brook, Illinois. This sponsorship reflects the Foundation's continuing international interest, which has spanned forty years, in hospital and health administration and education.

Conference participants represented government, universities, health care management (hospitals, public health planning agencies, and long-term care facilities), health policy, medical education, private foundations, national health associations and societies, and hospital-support industries. Papers were invited from a broad range of health industry leaders and others concerned with the education of health care managers; there was an attempt to address all major facets of the subject.

The objectives of the Conference were: to learn of the progress in implementing the Commission's recommendations; to informally critique, interpret, and discuss features and findings of the Commission's report; and to prepare a future agenda to advance education in health administration. Stimulated by nine very thoughtful papers, fruitful discussion included greater use of the university for continuing education and for nontraditional learning, the contribution of undergraduate education in health administration and its articulation with graduate programs, and enhancing the quality of education.

By the end of the two-day meeting many new and exciting ideas had emerged and much useful sharing had occurred. Exchanges and discussions tended to validate the Commission's findings and generally to support its recommendations. A set of strategies and a future agenda had emerged.

During the years since the Commission completed its study and issued its report, significant progress has been made, including: recent Foundation commitments for the establishment of external degree programs in health administration in the United States, and Canada; initiation of part-time and executive development programs for administrators who hold full-time health management positions; inauguration of a multi-university regional consortium to implement the Commission's recommendations; and renewed attention to the development of long-term care administrators and their professional society.

Finally, it should be noted that few professions have grown and developed as rapidly as health care administration. There is great demand for improvement in health care management, and the expectations of physicians and other health professionals, the government, insurance companies, the business community, and the public at large require that considerable progress be assured in the years ahead. While the health industry has faced tremendous changes and challenges, especially since 1965, we must anticipate even greater alterations in the delivery of, and payment for, health care in the next decade. To deal constructively with all of these issues a sound future agenda for education in health care administration is essential. The Conference gave us much hope for this and identified opportunities for improvement in the preparation of health care management practitioners. Much has been accomplished; much remains to be done. What will be your contribution?

ROBERT A. DeVRIES
Program Director

W. K. Kellogg Foundation
Battle Creek, Michigan

I

Rallying National Effort
to Improve
Health Administration Education

Karl D. Yordy: On behalf of myself, Nathan Stark, the Kellogg Foundation and many others, specifically George Bugbee, who has been so involved in arranging this conference, I would like to welcome you here. Many people have contributed, and I won't try to acknowledge them all now. Many of them are participating in the program. The theme of this conference, stated in rather grandiloquent terms, is "Rallying national effort to improve health administration education." The long and continued effort of the Kellogg Foundation in education for health administration has been expressed in recent times by its support of the Commission on Education for Health Administration (CEHA), many of whose members, including its Chairman, Dr. Dixon, are here with us. This conference is in many ways an extension of the Commission, its activities, and its report.

The purposes of the conference were stated briefly in the letters of invitation. We are here to consider the challenge faced by education for health administration, to review the recommendations of the Commission, to clarify and supplement those recommendations, to try to suggest new ideas for the improvement of the education of health administrators, and to create a sense of momentum that may have an impact on the field. The people invited are a diverse group, representing the educational community. Many of you use the products of education for health administration. Some are concerned with education more broadly and education policy

1

more broadly; some with health policy; and some with health administration and its practice and content.

I should mention two other activities that grew out of the Commission. The Kellogg Foundation appointed two task forces to specify means for implementing two of the Commission's recommendations—the development of one or more Centers for Advanced Study in Health Administration, and the planning of a program of lifelong learning and nontraditional study in the field. Members of both task forces, one headed by Nathan Stark and the other by myself, are here. Both task forces are in midstream in their deliberations, and there are interconnections between their studies and the subjects on this program. The task forces are in a position to benefit from the activities of this conference, but we are focusing on a number of issues that extend beyond the activities of the task forces. With those introductory comments on our purpose here, it is my now pleasure to introduce someone who has been very much involved in this field over a long period of time.

Andrew Pattullo: I have been looking forward to this meeting for a long time. It's an unusual kind of conference in one respect, in that I would guess that not everybody in this room knows everybody else, and I think that's good. It's a blending of people who come from health administration education, the field of practice, and government—all of whom are interested in the improvement of health.

Someone suggested that in my comments to you I might talk about the history of health administration education, and I decided not to do that. For one thing, I don't know that much about it, and secondly, I don't think you'd care that much about it. Instead, I'd like to give you some sort of a grasp of the Foundation's concern and involvement, and very deep interest, in the subject. The interest dates back almost 50 years, to when we were supporting a broad program for improving the quality of life in rural areas in southwest Michigan. A few of you here tonight, like Dr. Dixon, had a very real part in that campaign. During it we became quite aware of the deficiencies in the organization and management of health, as

2

well as in education and in other elements of community life. We became cognizant then of a need to develop some more formal method of preparing people for careers in the administration of health services.

As we look at the problems that we have as a nation today, that was a rather innocent era. Yet, in a way, it wasn't that innocent. In the early 1940s, education for health administration was almost completely in schools of public health, and it related to the administration of public health services for a broader community. There were two programs that were related to the administration of institutions, those of the University of Chicago and Northwestern University. Again, the problems of that time were much different from those of today, but there was very little ability on the part of the educational system to meet those needs. So, we became involved at that time in the development of programs of education for health administration, and in the ensuing three decades how that whole scene has changed! The educational establishment, the number of programs that are involved in health administration education, their location in the academic community, the diversity of graduate and undergraduate programs, programs that have an interest in a specialty organization such as long-term care. I don't recall the number of programs that are affiliated with the Association of University Programs in Health Administration, but I think it's something like 65 or 70, and that represents only a small proportion of the total. That's the educational side of it. Then you look at the programs in public health, or health of the public, and how the programs are responding to that need. It's a different view, a different setting, but it's still very much with us.

One further comment regarding the Foundation, which has had this long-standing concern for several decades. We entered into it with a conviction that there was a job to be done. Today we still have that conviction, that there is a need, and that educational programs for health administration have a very real role and opportunity to respond to that need. The mission of this conference is to look at the need, not in the sense of saving the world—I'm sure that's not going to happen—but we may take a few steps toward salvation, trying

3

to solve some of the problems that relate to why we're here. On behalf of the Foundation, we're grateful that so many have come here, and I express our special appreciation to Karl Yordy, Nathan Stark, and George Bugbee, and to Bob DeVries of the Foundation staff, for planning this program and putting it together. I have a feeling we're going to have a great time.

George Bugbee: The Foundation insisted that I be listed as coordinator, and I've been trying to think of what I might say that would justify both the title and this prominence on the program. I must confess that I've been a Foundation watcher for many years—with slight larceny in my soul at times, but in good causes. Involvement with the group that really built this program has been very pleasant for me.

Years ago, we brought together the secretaries of the state hospital associations to exhort them to perform more effectively. One of the sessions was about their problems, and a man whom I recall very well but who shall be nameless got up and said, "Now here is the problem: First I write the president's speech, and then I write the treasurer's report, and then the reports for the council chairmen. And when my turn comes, I can't think of anything I've done!" That doesn't quite apply to me, but there are a lot of people who have done the work for this program.

II

Current Status of Education
for Health Administration

Charles J. Austin, Ph.D.: The field of health administration education has grown rapidly from early beginnings characterized by a small number of vocationally-oriented programs in hospital administration and public health administration to a present position of maturity among the academic disciplines of our colleges and universities.[1] The rapid development of this educational specialty should not be surprising when one considers the complexity of the problems which beset our system for delivery of health care. The need for highly educated executives to provide leadership for the system becomes more evident every day.

The complexity of the health administrator's task can be seen in Figure II-1, which depicts the health administration process in open systems terms. Those involved in the administration of hospitals, medical clinics, long-term care facilities, mental health units, public health agencies, and similar organizations are overseeing an intricate process in which a varied set of inputs is converted to specific services to clients. Inputs to the conversion process include: assessment of needs and demands for health services; resources required for the provision of services (capital and operating funds, manpower, materials, and technology); consideration of community values; formal regulations imposed by external authorities; and "power inputs" (political positions which sometimes enhance and sometimes constrain the efficient provision of health services). The administrator must possess not only the necessary knowledge and skills for managing the internal operations of his organization; he also must be cognizant of those

5

FIGURE II-1

Health Administration Viewed as an Open System

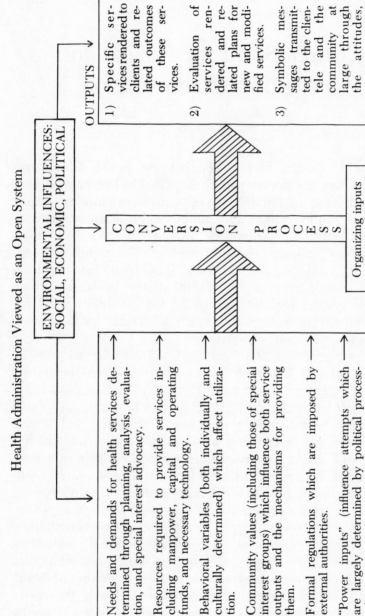

ENVIRONMENTAL INFLUENCES: SOCIAL, ECONOMIC, POLITICAL

INPUTS

→1) Needs and demands for health services determined through planning, analysis, evaluation, and special interest advocacy.

→2) Resources required to provide services including manpower, capital and operating funds, and necessary technology.

→3) Behavioral variables (both individually and culturally determined) which affect utilization.

→4) Community values (including those of special interest groups) which influence both service outputs and the mechanisms for providing them.

→5) Formal regulations which are imposed by external authorities.

→6) "Power inputs" (influence attempts which are largely determined by political processes).

→7) Administrative invention (spontaneity and creativity).

CONVERSION PROCESS

Organizing inputs into a set of formal and informal procedures for the delivery of services.

OUTPUTS

1) Specific services rendered to clients and related outcomes of these services.

2) Evaluation of services rendered and related plans for new and modified services.

3) Symbolic messages transmitted to the clientele and the community at large through the attitudes, gestures, and statements of those providing the services.

← FEEDBACK CYCLE →

external forces of the environment—social, economic, and political—within which the organization functions. Thus the process of health administration must be viewed through the dual lens of internal management and policy analysis, with both components heavily influenced by social, economic, and political factors.[2]

The difficulty of the administrative task is complicated even further by the economic scenario which our country faces for the next decade and beyond. All indications point to a continuing slowdown in economic growth, caused by several factors. We are becoming more and more aware of the scarcity of our natural resources, particularly energy resources. The economy has shifted from predominantly goods-producing to predominantly service-producing during the 25-year period since 1950. Since service industries are labor-intensive, slowdown in productivity increases necessarily follows. Environmental pressures also contribute to reduction in economic output. Finally, the redistribution of the age composition of the population results in a smaller ratio of productive workers to total population.

As the economy grows more slowly, there are fewer *new resources* to distribute among the social programs of the country. Since it is always more difficult to redistribute existing resources than to distribute new ones, those involved in the delivery of health services will find it more difficult to find the funds for new or expanded programs.

In sum, political decisions will be made within the framework of a politics of retrenchment. And yet there is no indication that demands for improved and increased health services will diminish in the years ahead. All these factors make the job of the health administrator more difficult, and yet more critically important.

The current status of education for health administration must be viewed within this context of complexity. Students must be familiar not only with principles of management, but also with the social, economic, and political environment within which health delivery organizations operate.

This paper is designed to set the stage for the conference and to provide an overview of the topics which will be examined during the next two days. In the first section, a brief description of this educational field is presented, including: data on educational objectives; the organization and financing of educational programs; characteristics of faculty, students, and alumni; descriptions of curricula; and related activities in research, continuing education, and community service. The second section of the paper highlights some of the major issues which face educators in this field. These include questions of manpower supply and demand, educational quality, the content of educational programs, the organization and financing of education for health administration, the role of undergraduate programs, the relationship between educators and practitioners, and the university's role in continuing education.

A Profile of Health Administration Education

Health administration programs exist in a variety of settings in colleges and universities. Continuing education programs are offered by a large number of practitioner and trade associations as well. Unfortunately, there is no central source of information which covers all educational efforts in this field. Hence, the data which follow had to be pieced together from several sources. The presentation is not intended to be comprehensive or exact. However, the profile presented should be sufficient to provide a good overview of current activity.

Some of the data which follow were obtained from surveys conducted by the Commission on Education for Health Administration (CEHA) during academic year 1972-73. More current information was obtained from the Association of University Programs in Health Administration (AUPHA), the primary professional association of faculty members in this field. Data obtained from AUPHA include information from the annual membership surveys, data from the task force on undergraduate education, and preliminary data from the AUPHA project studying the health and behavioral science components of health administration curricula.

Table II-1 is a summary of stated educational objectives

8

of graduate and undergraduate programs in health administration. Graduate programs tend to view their primary objective as the entry-level preparation of professional health administrators with particular emphasis on the administrative generalist. Graduate programs are also interested in the transmission of philosophical values about health and health services delivery. Health services research is an objective of most of the graduate programs, as are consultation and technical assistance to community health agencies. The continuing education of practicing administrators is the final objective mentioned most frequently by the faculty of graduate programs.

TABLE II-1

Educational Objectives

GRADUATE PROGRAMS
1. Entry-level preparation of professional health administrators with emphasis on generalist administrators.
2. Transmission of philosophical values about health and health services delivery.
3. Health services research.
4. Consultation and technical assistance.
5. Continuing education of practicing administrators.

UNDERGRADUATE PROGRAMS
1. Entry-level preparation of professional health administrators.
   a. Emphasis on middle managers and specialist administrators, particularly in long-term care.
   b. Focus on local or regional administrative manpower needs.
2. Continuing education of practicing administrators.
3. Preparation of students for graduate education.

Source: Commission on Education for Health Administration surveys, (1972–73).

At the undergraduate level, there is also a major focus on the entry-level preparation of professional health administrators. However, several of the programs emphasize the training of middle managers and specialist administrators, with particular emphasis on long-term care administration. Un-

9

dergraduate programs also tend to focus on local or regional manpower needs, and several of them offer part-time study for those working in local health organizations. The undergraduate programs emphasize continuing education for practicing administrators. Several of them also state that the preparation of students for graduate study in this field is an objective.

Table II-2 summarizes the organization of graduate programs in the United States and Canada. In academic year 1972-73, Commission surveys indicated that there were ap-

TABLE II-2

Graduate Programs in Health Administration
(U.S. and Canadian)

Number of Operational Programs Identified	72
Number of Programs Responding to Survey	54
ORGANIZATIONAL LOCUS	
Schools of Public Health	41%
Schools of Medicine and Allied Health	20%
Schools of Business/Public Administration	20%
Graduate Schools	8%
Multidisciplinary	9%
Other	2%
PARENT INSTITUTION	
Public University	57%
Private University	43%
AGE OF PROGRAM	
0-5 years	30%
6-10 years	22%
11-15 years	8%
16-20 years	8%
Over 20 years	32%

Source: Commission on Education for Health Administration surveys, (1972-73).

proximately 72 operational graduate programs. These programs were located in schools of public health, schools of medicine and allied health, schools of business and public administration, as well as in graduate schools, multidisciplinary settings, and others. The programs were approximately evenly divided between public and independent universities. Thirty-two percent of the programs surveyed were over 20 years old, but another 30 percent were fewer than 5 years old.

Undergraduate education in this field is a newer phenomenon. As indicated in Table II–3, the Commission estimated that there were 27 operational programs in existence during the year 1972–73. At present, there are 13 undergraduate programs holding membership in AUPHA. The Director of the AUPHA Undergraduate Task Force estimates that there are 130 or more undergraduate programs either in operation or in the planning stages. The oldest undergraduate program awarded its first degrees in 1956.

TABLE II–3

Undergraduate Programs in Health Administration*
(U.S. only)

Number of Programs with Students Enrolled (1972–73)—CEHA Estimates	27
Programs Holding AUPHA Membership (1976)	13
Programs with AUPHA Membership Pending (1976)	6
Estimated Number of Programs in Operation or in Planning Stages (1976)	130
Parent Institution Public University	61%
Private University	39%

* Oldest undergraduate program awarded its first degrees in 1956.

Source: Commission on Education for Health Administration surveys, (1972–73) and AUPHA Undergraduate Task Force.

Table II–4 indicates the breadth of the curriculum at the graduate level. Required courses cover the fields of management and administrative studies, behavioral and social sciences, health sciences, and medical care organization, as well as quantitative methods, planning, and other miscellaneous course work. Most of the programs require a formal field training period. Virtually all the programs require two years for completion of the master's degree.

The typical baccalaureate program (see Table II-5) includes approximately 50 percent of the curriculum in general education courses, 25 percent in health administration courses, with the remaining courses related to health administration subjects such as management, accounting, and allied health. Undergraduate programs also require a field training component, usually a summer internship of one to three months.

Faculty characteristics are summarized in Table II-6. Program facilities are small, with an average of 5.9 full-time faculty members in the graduate programs and 2.2 in the

TABLE II-4

Curricula: Graduate Programs
(U.S. and Canadian)

REQUIRED COURSES BY AREA OF STUDY	
Area	*Percent of all required courses*
Management/Administrative Studies	34
Behavioral/Social Sciences	21
Health Sciences	13
Medical Care Organization	10
Quantitative Methods	10
Miscellaneous	9
Planning	3

PREREQUISITE COURSES REQUIRED?	
Yes	40%
No	60%*

MOST COMMON PREREQUISITES (RANK ORDER)	
Economics	1
Accounting	2
Statistics	3

FIELD TRAINING REQUIRED?	
Yes	69%
No	31%

LENGTH OF FIELD TRAINING	
1–4 months	47%
5–8 months	16%
9–12 months	23%
Variable	14%

* Several of the programs which do not require undergraduate prerequisite courses actually include such courses in the first semester of the graduate curriculum.

Source: AUPHA Curriculum Project: a survey of 65 graduate programs including both AUPHA member programs and some nonmember programs.

TABLE II-5

Curricula: Undergraduate Programs
(U.S. only)

OVERALL CURRICULUM STRUCTURE	
Types of Courses	*Percent of Total Curriculum*
General Education Courses	46
Courses in Health Administration	24
Courses Related to Health Administration (Management, Allied Health, etc.)	30
FIELD TRAINING REQUIREMENTS	
1–3 Months	50
4–6 Months	13
Part-Time (Concurrent with On-Campus Study)	37

Source: Commission on Education for Health Administration surveys, (1972–73).

undergraduate programs. Sixty-one percent of the graduate program faculty members surveyed in 1972–73 held a doctorate degree compared to 37 percent for undergraduate faculty. Full-time faculty members in the graduate programs are

TABLE II-6

Faculty Characteristics.

	Graduate Programs*	Undergraduate Programs**
Average Number of Full-Time Faculty Members per Program	5.9	2.2
Average Number of Part-Time Faculty Members per Program***	8.2	3.3
Proportion of Full-Time Faculty Holding Doctorates	61%	37%
Proportion of Full-Time Faculty by Rank		
Professor	23%	
Associate Professor, Tenured	12%	
Associate Professor, Nontenured	13%	
Assistant Professor	33%	
Instructor	19%	

   * U.S. and Canadian graduate programs.

   ** Four-year baccalaureate programs only.

   *** Includes adjunct faculty appointments.

Source: Commission on Education for Health Administration surveys, (1972–73).

distributed across the four faculty ranks, with the preponderance at the lower ranks. The newer faculty members tend to be young men and women with strong academic training. While they bring an important conceptual base to their research and teaching, they lack experience in the operational problems that health organizations face.

There were approximately 3,900 graduate students enrolled in educational programs in health administration during academic year 1972–73, and an additional 600 students in undergraduate programs (see Table II–7). Women are still in

TABLE II-7

Student Enrollment Statistics

	GRADUATE PROGRAMS (U.S. AND CANADIAN)		
	AUPHA MEMBER AND ASSOCIATE MEMBER PROGRAMS		
Year	Number of Programs	Total Enrollment*	Average Number of Students per Program
1972	38	2185	58
1973	38	2154	57
1974	44	2236	51
CEHA SURVEYS (1972–73)			
Estimate of Total Number of Students Enrolled			3,900
Female Students			25%
Minority Students			12%
UNDERGRADUATE PROGRAMS (U.S. ONLY)			
CEHA SURVEYS (1972–73)			
Estimate of Total Number of Students Enrolled			600
Female Students			33%
Minority Students			14%

* First and second year students.

Sources: AUPHA Annual Membership Surveys and Commission on Education for Health Administration.

the minority, but increases have been noted in recent years. Approximately 12 percent of all students enrolled were members of ethnic minority groups. More recent data from the AUPHA membership surveys show a continuous increase in enrollment among the AUPHA member and associate member programs.

Data on the post-graduate experience of alumni are difficult to obtain. However, Commission surveys for the year 1972–73 indicate that approximately 2,100 graduate and 183 undergraduate degrees were awarded that year (see Table II–8). The limited data available on placements indicate that over one-half of the graduates at the master's level took positions as hospital administrators, and approximately 50 percent of the undergraduate alumni also assumed positions in hospitals. The AUPHA membership surveys indicate that there were 10,555 graduate program alumni as of December 31, 1974.

TABLE II-8

Program Graduates

CEHA Surveys (1972-73)	Graduate Programs	Undergraduate Programs
Degrees Awarded	2,100	183
Most Common Placement (5% or more)		
a. Hospital Administration	53%	48%
b. Government Health Agencies	13%	—
c. Health Planning Agencies	5%	9%
d. Long-Term Care Administration	—	10%
e. Ambulatory Care Administration	5%	—
f. Further Study	—	20%
AUPHA Membership Surveys		
Degrees Awarded		
1972	899	
1973	970	
1974	1,005	
Total Number of Alumni as of December 31, 1974	10,555	

Finally, Table II-9 documents some of the related program activities at the graduate level. Twenty percent of the graduate-program faculty time is spent in research, and about 27 percent of the program budgets from all sources (including grants and contracts) is devoted to research. Continuing education takes on lesser importance, with 8 percent of the faculty's time and 4 percent of the program budgets devoted to this activity. Sixty-five percent of the programs have formal community service programs of technical assistance to local health agencies and institutions.

This brief profile can describe the field only in very general terms. For more detail, the reader is directed to the paper "Education for Health Administration: A Statistical Profile" in Volume II of *Education for Health Administration*.[3]

TABLE II-9

Related Program Activities

GRADUATE PROGRAMS (U.S. AND CANADIAN)	
Percent of Faculty Time Devoted to Research	20
Percent of Faculty Time Devoted to Continuing Education	8
Percent of Program Budgets* Devoted to Research	27
Percent of Program Budgets* Devoted to Continuing Education	4
Percent of Programs with Formal Community Service Programs (e.g., Technical Assistance)	65

* Funds from all sources, including grants and contracts.
Source: Commission on Education for Health Administration Surveys, (1972–73).

Major Educational Issues

The directors and faculty of educational programs in this field are confronted by most of the general problems facing higher education during a period of retrenchment. However, this section of the paper describes more specific issues which often are debated by those involved in health administration programs. The issues are raised but not joined. They will be more completely explored in subsequent discussions.

Manpower Supply and Demand

There is considerable controversy and confusion among educators and practicing administrators over questions of manpower supply and demand. The pessimistic view suggests that the field is being over-supplied with new graduates and predicts that the manpower market will become glutted in the years ahead. The opposite view holds that there will be many new health programs developed as the result of government activity and other forces at work in the system, and that these new programs will provide virtually unlimited opportunities for trained manpower in the next decade or so.

Unfortunately, there is no good information system on which to base manpower projections for health administrators. One of the few analytical studies is that by Feldman and Rossett. Their findings indicate that the supply and demand for hospital administrators will remain in approximate balance during the years immediately ahead, provided there is no rapid increase in supply beyond that which has occurred in recent years.[4] When one moves beyond the field of hospital administration, it is much more difficult to estimate future manpower requirements. Some have argued that the development of new programs will continue to provide ample opportunities for program graduates. Others take the position that there is a fixed administrative overhead available to organizations involved in the delivery of health services and that the demand for administrators is not unlimited; i.e., the percentage of Gross National Product devoted to health care will determine the number of administrative positions to be filled, regardless of how services are organized.

The apparent disparity between job market conditions and student market conditions in this field is a related and important issue for educators. If, in fact, the job market is tightening, what is the societal obligation of colleges and universities to assess job opportunities and to constrain their student recruiting activities—despite heightened student interest?

Finally, there is general agreement among health administration educators that continued efforts should be made to attract qualified women and members of ethnic minority groups to the field.

Educational Quality

Specific measures of educational quality are the subject of debate in this field, as in higher education generally. There appear to be no good outcome or impact measures by which educational quality can be evaluated; hence, the current measures of quality center on structure and process.

17

The role of program accreditation in promoting educational quality is a hotly debated topic. Many faculty members believe that program accreditation has been the single most important factor in upgrading graduate programs and in promoting higher levels of educational quality. Others tend to minimize the value of the accreditation process.

The relatively small size of educational programs in this field was noted earlier. Some have argued that there is a minimum level of resources required to provide a high quality educational program and that many of the existing programs are too small and have inadequate resources. The proponents of this view argue for a smaller number of larger programs. A counter-argument suggests that the size of the program is not as important as the total resource base which can be effectively used by faculty and students. Thus, the extent of inter- and intra-university relationships becomes the most important question in considering the quality of an educational program.

Fortunately, the debate over organizational locus (i.e., whether the program *must* be located in a school of public health or *must* be located in a school of management) seems to have been laid to rest. There is general agreement that a good program can be developed in a variety of settings, provided that university-wide resources are accessible to the program.

Another important issue related to educational quality is the shortage of qualified faculty members available for university programs. Faculty members have a diversity of backgrounds, ranging from senior people with considerable operating experience to younger ones with good academic training in a discipline but with little direct operating experience. Although some programs are heavily involved in health services research, there is concern about the overall level and quality of the research. Since research is closely related to curriculum quality, the need to stimulate improved research activity is an important educational issue.

The Content of Educational Programs

A major question among educators is the generalist versus specialist issue. Should educational programs be preparing generalist health administrators with broad knowledge of the complex needs of the health care system? Or should the administrative task be subdivided for solution by functional specialists in such areas as finance, planning, and human resources? Alternatively, should we train categorical specialists who understand the specific environments of hospitals, or nursing homes, or medical health institutions, or public health agencies? Still another point of view argues for the education of the generalist administrator with a specific disciplinary skill—to provide an analytic basis for integrating multidisciplinary approaches to problem solving.

A second major issue related to educational content is the question of the field training component of the curriculum. Several programs have adopted a two-year academic format, while others have retained a one-year administrative residency. Debate continues about the efficacy of each approach.

There is still some debate about whether the curriculum of a program should reflect a health orientation or a management orientation. However, the field seems to have matured to the point at which there is general recognition of the need for a conceptual, problem-solving approach. Earlier debate about the proper orientation of a program derived from a narrower and more descriptive view of the educational process. The complexity of the administrative process as described earlier in this paper presents strong argument for the analytical approach.

Finally, a major concern of those involved in curriculum planning is the increased involvement of government and other regulatory agencies in the health care system. This has generated increased attention to the need for policy analysis in the curriculum of educational programs in this increasingly public field.

Organization and Financing of Education
for Health Administration

A crucial issue facing faculty members in this field is the willingness, or unwillingness, of university administrators to provide a base level of support for their programs during times of economic retrenchment. A related question is the need for federal support, if any. Faculty research efforts have been hampered by the generally low level of federal funding available for studies in health services organization, planning, and delivery.

David Starkweather has presented strong arguments supporting the value of an effective infrastructure among educational programs in this field.[5] The appropriate role of the Association of University Programs in Health Administration in this regard needs further study and definition.

A more recent issue is the increasing state regulation of educational programs by coordinating boards of higher education. What will be the effects of such regulation on the development of new programs and on the continuation of existing programs in health administration?

Finally, the need for doctoral programs to produce teachers and researchers in health services administration is an important question. Given the need for these programs, is the resource base of existing university programs adequate to provide the advanced levels of research and teaching which are essential to effective doctoral studies?

Educator-Practitioner Relationships

There is concern among many health administration practitioners regarding the lack of administrative experience of younger faculty members. While these faculty members bring an essential conceptual base to their teaching and research, they need a better blend of theoretical skills and operating experience. A suggested solution is more involvement of faculty in consultation, technical assistance, and applied research.

Many practitioners are also concerned about the demise of the administrative residency in a large proportion of the academic programs. Practitioners seem to believe that the residency is still an important part of the development of a fledgling administrator.

Finally, there is concern about the widening gap between professional associations and educators in health services administration. The "town and gown" conflict has accelerated in recent years, and many educators are striving for more effective communications and relationships with their counterparts in the field of practice.

The Role of Undergraduate Education

Debate abounds concerning the appropriate role, if any, of undergraduate education in health administration. A major question centers on the available job market for graduates of undergraduate programs. Some have suggested middle management and specialist administrator positions. Others argue quite effectively for the preparation of generalist administrators at the undergraduate level.

The basic question of whether articulation between undergraduate and graduate programs is possible or desirable has yet to be resolved. Some graduate-level educators believe that a broad undergraduate preparation in the liberal arts and behavioral sciences is more appropriate for entry into graduate-level programs than is specialized education in the field of health administration. The question of job articulation is also important. Is there truly a job progression in the health administration field so that individuals can move up as they advance their education?

Among undergraduate educators a basic question is which fundamental approach to follow in curriculum design. Should the approach consist of a general liberal arts education, with health administration providing a set of problems to which the liberal arts can be applied? Or should the curriculum follow the professional school model and provide a more technical education?

The University's Role in Continuing Education

Considerable attention is being focused on continuing education in this field, partly as a result of the findings of the Commission on Education for Health Administration which

21

documented the needs for lifelong learning. An important issue for university educators concerns the appropriate role of the university in providing continuing education. Traditionally, university reward systems have provided little incentive for faculty members to engage in these activities. Questions about the appropriate level and amount of academic credit to be granted for continuing education courses must also be addressed.

Conclusion

This paper has attempted not to provide answers, but to raise fundamental questions which this conference needs to address. Its intent has been to provide an overview of the current status of education for health administration and its major issues.

Where is this educational field headed? In the opinion of the author, it is moving in the right direction. Faculties have been strengthened in recent years. Curricula have shifted from a descriptive, almost vocational, approach to a conceptual and analytical framework for advanced study. Important new funding sources are on the horizon, and research opportunities abound. Educators and practitioners are once again joining together to solve some of the problems which the system faces.

The directional signs are good, but the needs for strengthening programs are also well documented. The Commission on Education for Health Administration suggested several avenues for improvement. The deliberations of this conference could provide impetus and direction for implementing the Commission's recommendations.

Notes

[1] Charles J. Austin, Daniel A. Clark, and James A. Ball, "Education for Health Administration: A Statistical Profile," in *Education for Health Administration*, Vol. II (Ann Arbor: Health Administration Press, 1975), pp. 71–73.

[2] Charles J. Austin, "What is Health Administration?" *Hospital Administration*, Summer 1974, pp. 20–22.

[3] Austin, Clark, and Ball, op. cit., pp. 71–143.

[4] Roger Feldman and Richard N. Rossett, "The Demand for Hospital Administrators," *Education for Health Administration*, Vol. II (Ann Arbor: Health Administration Press, 1975), pp. 317–330.

[5] David B. Starkweather, "The Organizational Network of Education for Health Administration," in *Education for Health Administration*, Vol. II (Ann Arbor: Health Administration Press, 1975), pp. 317–330.

III

Current Developments Affecting Health Administration and the Role of the Health Administrator

William R. Roy, M.D., J.D.: I am very pleased to have the opportunity to participate in this conference on education for health administration. The Commission on Education for Health Administration (CEHA) has done an especially fine piece of work in this critical area, and it is fitting that efforts to implement as many of its recommendations as possible should begin immediately. This is especially true in view of the increasing demands on health administrators created by rapid change in the American health care system.

As I identify current developments affecting health administration and administrators, I am sure I will lapse into referring to past developments and possible future developments. Education is, I believe, preparation for dealing with change; not only change that we can currently observe or anticipate, but change that, today, we can not even imagine. For this reason, I was pleased to hear Dr. Austin speak of the conceptual and analytical emphasis in schools of health administration. And when I mentioned this to one of the finest health administrators I know, she agreed and added the word "think." We, the rest of society, are imposing great burdens on health administrators, and we are counting on you to help modify some problems that do not have wholly acceptable solutions.

In addition, it is my intention to play an advocacy role as I talk about current developments. I believe it is best to state my preferences flat out rather than to imply them, especially when many of you already know what they are. I will speak about the National Health Planning and Resources Development Act, the newest game in town (some people are flattering enough to refer to it as the only game in town), and other regulatory cost containment efforts. I will then refer briefly to health manpower legislation and efforts to organize health care services better. Throughout, I will emphasize my conviction that definitive regulation is inevitable, because health marketplace mechanisms are gone forever.

We have two major problems in the health field. The one receiving our immediate attention is cost containment. The other, which I will only touch upon today, is the evaluation of the many factors that determine health, most particularly personal health services—in other words, what we are getting in return for our expenditures.

We may or may not be spending too much for health today. But at least four forces—(1) patient expectations, (2) the technological imperative, (3) open-ended, third-party payment, and (4) a physician ethic to provide all health care to each patient—have caused the health care system to be described as a giant vacuum cleaner that will suck up all the dollars made available to it. Few, if any, within our society will contend that it is mathematically possible to continue indefinitely the current trends in increased expenditures for health, or that it is possible even in wealthy, modern America to do everything medically and scientifically possible for everyone, everywhere.

One result of this is that we are now implementing the Health Planning and Resources Development Act in an effort to allocate limited resources intelligently. This law requires the regulation of capital expenditures, because capital expenditures are required to build and equip facilities in which health services are provided. Each state must implement a certificate of need law, and a certificate of need must be obtained before the capital expenditure can be made. The planning law provides for a Health Systems Agency to review the capital expenditure proposal and to recommend its approval or disapproval, based on whether or not the improvement is consistent with a five-year health systems plan, and with an annual implementation plan for providing health services to the people of an identified geographic area. Successful implementation of this law will require a skilled staff for the Health Systems Agency. Competence of the staff and the agency will probably be the most significant factor in the success or failure of each HSA. The designated state agency will have similar staff requirements.

For those traditional health administrators, the hospital administrators, the new law will provide new requirements and challenges. Hospitals and other health institutions must plan well if they are to compete. Institutional plans must be consistent with state health plans and health service area plans. Ad hoc ventures that are not foreseen will be unlikely to get certificates of need. There will be a new role for the hospital board, and new relationships among administration, board, and medical staff. While plans will be subject to annual revisions, an institution's future mission will be substantially directed when the first health systems plan is written.

For many of us, the health planning law as presently constituted is only the beginning. Because we are convinced that input regulation as represented by facility and health services planning is the most rational and satisfactory form of regulation, it makes good sense to me that people within localities and states decide what health services they want, need, and are willing to pay for. Parenthetically, these are not the same things. My support of the health planning law is based on the conclusion that regulation is inevitable, because there is no other way to control costs. Let me try to convince you—if it is necessary—that a definitive regulatory mechanism (or mechanisms) is necessary.

In the free enterprise system, the marketplace is the traditional and most efficient method of allocating services. In health, the marketplace has been destroyed over the last 40 years by health insurance. It can be restored only by passing a law prohibiting health insurance. This will not happen for many reasons, including the size of medical bills, the concept that health care is a right, and the popularity of health insurance. In fact, the last remnants of a marketplace will be destroyed by the passage of universal, mandatory, national health insurance. So we can praise the marketplace, the laws of supply and demand, the free enterprise system, and personal responsibility to prepare for a rainy day, but for health care, these are all gone. I do not rejoice, nor do I mourn; I simply recognize this fact of life.

We may experiment for a while with modified market mechanisms in an effort to contain health costs, but most of these too will pass. Copayments, coinsurance, and deductibles will not work, because the American people will buy first-dollar supplementary health insurance as long as the law allows it. Moreover, both the limitation of the benefit package and the mechanisms of copayment, coinsurance, and deductibles distort the system. A restricted-payment mechanism puts health insurers and legislators in the business of making medical decisions, because reimbursability effectively determines not only who will get services but also who will provide services, what services will be provided, and where they will be provided.

There is one market mechanism that may have limited success. Large buyers of health services may be able to bargain with large providers of services for prices and numbers of services. But this gross mechanism will mature too late to head off universal, mandatory, comprehensive, first-dollar health insurance. However, if we are careful about our legislative initiative, such efforts will not be incompatible with national health insurance and other changes in the health system.

I have ruled out consumer incentives for containing costs. We also hear a lot about provider incentives, such as those that are said to operate in an HMO. Let me say that as I understand provider incentives, they are not incompatible with most concepts of national health insurance, and they may be used to encourage efficiency, but in this age of great consumer demand and the technological imperative, they are not going to contain costs substantially. So like it or not, politically popular or not, public utility-like or not, we are going to be regulated. The only question is how.

One effort—around for a long time but only now being implemented—is the combination of utilization review and Professional Standards Review Organizations. I do not believe these efforts are going to do much to contain costs, although I believe PSROs are a much needed complementary regulation for quality control, and that utilization review must continue to minimize potential gross abuses of open-ended, third-party payments.

A third mechanism for controlling cost is an arbitrary determination by third-party payers of how much they will spend for health services. These arbitrary limitations are usually called "caps." Government caps are determined on one basis only—how much the government is willing to pay. Caps are notoriously unrelated to demand or to need, or even to the number of services rendered. And caps are characteristically unrelated to the cost of services. Many adverse effects result from this most recent development in Medicaid in many states, and from this recommended method for Medicare cost containment. These adverse results include: (1) an irrational curtailment of services; (2) a shift of institutional costs to other government services or to private services; (3) a widening of the dual system of government payment for the poor, disabled, and aged, and private payment for all others; (4) the withdrawal of services by physicians; and (5) oftentimes greater costs than would be incurred if services were fully reimbursable in a variety of settings. For example, some patients are forced to receive services in teaching-hospital outpatient departments at a much higher cost than if the same services were rendered in a private physician's office. Health administrators, as I know them, both implement government caps and struggle with the effects of government caps. And both are happening today.

Another regulatory effort affecting health administration today is the creation of state hospital commissions. These have shown promise, and the National Health Planning and Resources Development Act provides federal funding for six of them. The most promising mechanism is prospective budgeting, whereby budgets for the fiscal year are submitted for review and approval. It was recognized at the time the Health Planning Act was written that rate regulation, ser-

28

vices development, and planning must be coordinated efforts; that services provided in an approved and developed facility must be paid for if planning is to have any meaning; and that quality of services must be maintained. Conversely, it was realized that services available and reimbursable would probably be utilized, and that not only capital costs but operating costs must be considered in planning and granting certificates of need. It is my hope that amendments to the law will provide for both the coordination and balance of these closely associated regulatory functions. Health administrators will continue to administer and contend with rate regulation, most desirably as a part of the planning and development of services.

Finally, as a warning, permit me to remind you that wage and price controls are a real possibility for what is called the "health industry." Congress and the Administration have wage and price control for health under continuous consideration. I am personally convinced that this is inherently bad regulation, for two reasons: it has all the adverse effects of arbitrary caps, and, in the absence of control over related industries, it is destined to fail over a period of time. But health administrators must always be aware that wage and price controls are a favored government regulatory mechanism. These controls are particularly admired by those unfamiliar with the intricacies of the health system—a system peculiar in that certain people are entitled to services by law and by private third-party payment—factors which do not affect most commodities and industries.

I have expressed a strong preference for planning and developing the health system and services on the local and state level. I have spoken of this as "input regulation." But the control of facilities is only one part of input regulation. The other is determining numbers and kinds of manpower, because facilities plus manpower equals services. Facilities cannot provide services without manpower and, in modern health care, few health professionals can provide services without facilities. Personal health services are one determinant of health. Services are what we want, and of course services are what we pay for. Under national health insurance, all or

29

nearly all services will be paid for, and our experience shows that paid-for health services will be used. Therefore, the least unsatisfactory and least rigid way that I can conceive of for rationally controlling services and costs is limiting services by limiting inputs (facilities and manpower). I reiterate that we should do this on the basis of what the American people want, need, and are willing to pay for. Therein lies the challenge of getting the American people to participate in planning and in other activities, so that they can express what they want, need, and are willing to pay for.

To return to the subject of health manpower, given the facilities, health care providers (especially physicians) can create demand. This is not an accusation that physicians do this consciously or purposefully. For the most part, physicians treat patients the way they were trained to treat patients. A gastroenterologist trained in endoscopy treats patients with gastrointestinal complaints differently from the way the family physician or general internist treats patients with the same complaints. Another way of saying this is, *Given only a hammer, the whole world looks like a nail.*

The new health manpower proposals would limit and reapportion residency positions among the specialties. This has strong service implications for health administrators whose institutions have provided—and perhaps are expected to continue to provide—certain services whose manpower component consists of physicians in training. Moreover, the new manpower proposals will make more physicians available for presently underserved areas, which means relatively fewer physicians available for areas with currently high physician populations.

Finally, a limitation of services, perhaps ultimately determined by facility limitations (capital expenditure regulation, i.e., health planning) and manpower training decisions, will affect health administrators in other ways. With universal entitlement and high demand, one can anticipate a gatekeeping function for some administrators at some places. On a more optimistic note, one can expect a more intense and more efficient use of facilities and services, and better education of the public in the use of health services. Both imply additional roles for health administrators in cooperation with other health professionals. All these consequences, plus present problems, require health administrators to work with others in finding better organizational methods for providing health services. HMO management and other group practice management, foundation management, hospital outpatient management, primary care group practice management—and a thousand other areas—cry out for more effective and more efficient ways of providing quality health services.

I have talked a lot about planning the system and planning the services. Planning is a good idea, and it is necessary. But it is very difficult to do well today, and it would be difficult to do well even if the structure and process for doing so were fully in place. The reason is that we have so little data and such great gaps in required information. We often do not know the health benefits of the things we do, and it is not possible to measure *cost benefits* if we don't know the *benefits*. So there is an immediate need for more and better data, a monitoring of what we are doing, and satisfactory evaluation plans for the things we intend to do.

Again, I do not know the specific role for that protean person known as the *health administrator* in this area, but I know that there is a role, and that there will be an increasing number of roles for the administrator in all these efforts. I am certain that I have overlooked many current developments that affect health administration and health administrators, but, after all, you who are health administrators feel them, and for the most part I only think about them. I hope I have touched upon a few of the most important developments, and that I have to some degree provided a feeling for the direction of future developments.

Comment

James P. Dixon, M.D.: I liked the metaphor about the hammer and the nail. As you were talking, I was trying to figure out where the health administrator feels *he* is. I expect he may think that he's the nail and regulation is the hammer. I'd like to examine one or two of the trends that have been discussed and see if that might help us work out what makes sense in the formal training of health administrators. I find myself in the position of having a rather intense dislike of the mechanism of regulation. So let me overcome that by saying that there are a couple of trends that underline what has been said— trends that, in a way, lie outside the health field. If we are talking about rationalizing the field, and about the educational institution as a means of putting theory to data and of handling the rationalizing of a situation, we have a circumstance in which the left and right fringes of the intellectual community are in agreement. It is probably true that the fringes of a community influence the possibilities for change, and that the middle provides the inertia against change. For a long time the left fringe of the intellectual community has strongly argued for decentralization. It has become an article of faith that the management of human services should be returned, in some fashion, closer to the community; that this is where planning should occur; and that this is where certain kinds of crucial decisions should be made, in order to mitigate both the natural variations that exist across the country and the problem of resources. It now happens that the intellectual right takes the same position, a position strongly opposed to the heavy centralization of activities in a bureaucracy. In higher education the monopoly is moving toward the states, with an effort to see whether the state can provide some mechanism to put on the caps and to implement other controls. Within the universities, it seems likely that there will be support for some mechanism which pushes control back toward the local community; but it seems unlikely that there will be support for the regulatory mechanism.

It may be that the universities are the last bastion of laissez faire. The practice of medicine comes fairly close to being a bastion of laissez faire, but the universities are *the* last bastion. There will be real difficulty, it seems to me, in developing a theoretical construct which is satisfactory for the development of this kind of planned

32

service economy in the health field. I'm inclined to think that one measure of success with respect to this trend will be whether or not people who move into health service administrative roles can, in fact, cooperate with public policy in ways which convert physicians into mercenaries. It seems to me that in a highly regulated or planned economy the professionalization of civil servants goes up and the professionalization—the autonomy—of the professions goes down. One question we can ask ourselves is, do we have ways of dealing with educational strategy that will in fact change the balance of power between the health administrator and the professional? Will there be a reinforcement of the administrator's ability to enforce the behavior of the professional, on whatever grid and controlled by whatever boundaries that public policy calls for?

As Dr. Roy was talking, I was reminded that in my halcyon days even some of the national trade associations thought they might think openly about the public utility concept—before the back of the system was broken, and it became inchoate. This suggests that the politics of this kind of planning are also going to be extremely complicated, and that the alliance of the health administrator with political groups will be an important factor in accomplishing this kind of organization.

Let me also say something more about the impact on education. While I realize that we are not here to hash over or to instruct the task groups that are working on the Commission report, I think it's interesting to reflect that there are two efforts being explored in education for health administration. One is the effort to see whether the analysis and intellectual effort which health administrators provide for the system can in some way be improved; this is partly a process of selection and partly a process of pedagogy. The second, however, seems almost to fit your trend model; it is a set of discussions of how one can effectively use the local community as a training arena. Can one use data from the local community as part of the curriculum for the preparation of

33

health administrators? If it is true that initiative is to be shifted to the local level and that this will increase (rather than decrease) the diversity of decisions in the face of rigid boundaries at a more general level, it seems that one needs to find out "where the action is" for the material that will be effective in training educators for the future.

One final comment—I suppose in the nature of an apologia for finding oneself in the position of agreeing with a disagreeable prospect. Some research on Social Security suggests that the more centralized the mechanism for the delivery of Social Security services, the larger the number of dollars that ends up with the consumer. If we look at the health field, what we appear to be saying is that this matter is going to be brought under control. Is there a nonviolent way of doing that? That's really the kind of question that's being raised. This does indicate that decentralization will probably reduce the amount of expenditure at the point of impact, which suggests to me that an understanding of the micro-economics of health services delivery may become very important to health service administrators; this in addition to the macro-economics which are implied by your notion of system. I find your discussion very provocative.

Discussion

Charles C. Edwards M.D. (presiding): I too am convinced that whether we like it or not, regulation is inevitable, and if we don't contain costs, then I think the ultimate answer is fairly obvious. One of the problems that we who have been looking at the administrators (particularly we of the federal health care system) have failed to recognize is that we have asked the Department of Health, Education, and Welfare to do things that it can't do, and couldn't do even if it were staffed appropriately. We've asked HEW staff members to be program managers, and I think they have been, with reasonable success. We've also asked them to be regulators, and if you look at the record of HEW as a regulator, it's disastrous. Dr. Roy mentioned utilization review. We may mention PSRO, or we can talk about the end-stage renal disease program. All these are in a sense regulatory programs, in an environment in which the department is about as apolitical as possible, and I recognize the problems that go with that.

There's also the job that we have to begin to educate those who are not health professionals. My experience, and Ted Cooper's as Assistant Secretary at HEW, are probably as good as any I can think of. We had put together what we thought was a team of pretty good managers—some damn good administrators. We spent many months developing the so-called Forward Plan. We reviewed it with members of Congress, and they thought it was great. In informal conversations we reviewed it with members of the Office of Management and Budget, who were intrigued with the concept. But when push came to shove, apparently because of lack of confidence in the health care administrators at HEW, Congress went to the Harvard Business School types at OMB and totally ignored our recommendations. My point is very simple: there is certainly a lack of confidence out there in many of us who are involved in the field of health care administration.

Let me make a side comment on the need to have a control organization such as a National Health Authority. To me, the need seems quite obvious. For instance, one of the things that concerns me right now about the Planning Act—and I couldn't agree more with Bill Roy that it's the only act in town, and I think we have to make it work—is that there's nothing that these Health Systems Agencies are going to have to relate to. They don't have a Federal Reserve Board, or anything within the federal structure. Not that I would like to see a group of people in Washington deciding what doctors are going to charge, what their fees are going to be, or exactly how hospitals are going to be reimbursed. But I think there has to be some central federal organization that provides guidelines and standards, and which gives a certain kind of direction that regional, state, and local groups have to use in their planning and implementation efforts.

Following Dr. Edwards's introductory comments, the discussion turned first to the woeful inadequacy of support for health service research and the consequent lack of data, understanding, and trained health care analysts. Funds for health service research amount to only .02 percent of aggregate health care expenditures. As expenditures for personal health services have gone up, expenditures for all other health service initiatives have gone down, due mainly to a lack of understanding in the Congress, where the view prevails that the only worthwhile research is that directed to specific problems such as cancer and heart disease. Health service research and statistics had high priority in HEW's Forward Plan, as Dr. Edwards reported, "We're not going to solve the problems we've been talking about here until we have that kind of information." The need for information, and especially the need for training specialists in health care analysis, can be met only if these activities are emphasized and supported in the universities, it was suggested.

The emphasis on the need for data evoked an iconoclastic objection: "I don't think the big problem is data," said a health economist. "We have lots of data, and any time we're short we can manufacture some. Lots of our data are good, but the big problem is a conceptualization of data. What is it that we want the data for? We need to think about the purposes in order to know what kind of data we want. If you try to get data for all possible purposes, you will just get swamped, and you'll never have time to look at any of it."

A related problem is the need to train more qualified personnel for public service. One of the problems with regulation of the health services is that most regulators have been trained in government, but not in health services. "We need health administration graduates in the public health departments, but we can't get them," one participant said. Another suggested that the training of health service regulators should be a specific responsibility of the universities.

"We tend to forget who employs health administrators," a university representative noted. "The balance of power can't be understood without recognizing the difference between opportunities for health administrators employed in the industry and the small number of those with direct public responsibility. This has implications for education. We shouldn't give students objectives they can't achieve."

Another program director saw the training of regulators and the development of theories about regulation as an exciting opportunity for the universities. The issue of state as opposed to federal roles in planning and regulation, and the introduction of federal-state shared responsibility without clarifying either role (as in Public Law 93-641), should be a fascinating subject for investigation.

Dr. Roy acknowledged that the effort to get more specific authority for regulation into the Planning Act had failed. "We would have had rate regulation if I'd had my way," he said. "There was an effort to decentralize control, but not enough money to pay the states for what the federal government wants them to do. There was to have been a single agency for planning, capital expense regulation, or resource development, and rate regulation, but it didn't work out that way, although control of capital expense, at least, is at the state level. As it has turned out, there is no coordination among the three lines of control, and rate regulation can negate planning and capital control."

Dr. Edwards concluded the discussion by pointing out that we've had both successes and failures in regulation:

Whenever you talk about regulation those who are anti-regulation bring up the failures and not the successes. If you look at our federal regulatory efforts, there may be more failures than successes, but there are some successes. And it behooves us to find a way to regulate, because it's inconceivable that we can carry the system much further without regulation. I believe that you can regulate if you structure a regulatory system that takes the regulators as far away from the day-to-day political environment as possible. You can't be a regulator in HEW when you've got the Congress hitting you on one side, the president and the Office of Management and Budget hitting you on the other, and masses of special interest groups hitting you on the third side, as does the FDA Commissioner. You can't regulate in an environment like that. You have to have some protection. I believe you can develop an organizational structure that could conceivably work. Again, if it doesn't work, what are the options?

IV

Unmet Needs in Education
for Health Administration

Lawrence A. Hill: In approaching this assignment I was immediately struck by two thoughts, neither of which is very complimentary to the planners of this conference. The first may be semantic and I mention it only to demonstrate that there remains some academic snobbery in my makeup. The title, *Unmet Needs*, seems to me to be a redundancy. Once a need is met it is no longer a need. Thus a need is by definition unmet.

The second thought is far more important and goes to the heart of this presentation. The other papers will deal with the financing of education, undergraduate education, improving the content in education, and achieving quality in education. It would seem that if all those subjects were successfully addressed by the academic community, there would be few if any needs left to meet. In a sense, then, the entire conference deals with needs. Therefore I reached something of an impasse, because each thought I generated was someone else's assignment. At first I was irritated, and then I realized that George Bugbee was challenging me to think a little. He knows how difficult that is for me. Accordingly, I decided to try to address this topic in a manner which could contain some value, if for no other reason than that it might provoke some discussion here, and which might even provoke further discussion among faculty members in their own institutions and in their own professional associations.

Using the first two volumes of *Education for Health Administration* and some personal thoughts, or prejudices, as texts, I identified two areas of need which I believe have not

39

been well-addressed by educators in health administration. These are, first, a lack of market orientation and a better definition of market demand for graduates, and second, the production of scholars and teachers in the field. The two needs are related. Both needs relate to a gap between the fields of academia and practice. I will first comment on the production of scholars and then turn to the market.

Production of Scholars and Teachers

During the years in which graduate studies in health administration were being formulated, teachers in health administration came primarily from two sources. They were either hospital administrators or practitioners of public health. Because of their practice-oriented approach, curricula tended to be descriptive of current practices rather than analytic. Teaching tended to be located in the field as much or more than in the classroom. Students were chosen who had already demonstrated an interest in, and who had had some actual experience in, health services administration or, in some cases, in the provision of clinical services.

As with most concepts, the results were both good and bad. On the positive side, there emerged from these programs a group of graduates who were highly motivated and practice-oriented and whose frame of reference had probably been substantially broadened and deepened during their educational experience. In addition, the programs served as a credentialing mechanism. The M.P.H. soon became an important credential in public health departments, and the M.H.A. or equivalent degree began replacing the F.A.C.H.A. (awarded by the American College of Hospital Administrators) as the key hospital credential. Especially in hospital administration, because of the high demand for positions, the graduate programs became screening devices, which undoubtedly served to recruit better candidates, and by implication weeded out those who were not so good. In short, the practitioner-teacher model did fulfill a definite purpose and demonstrated the value of formal preparation for health service administrators. This model, however, had some drawbacks, which became more and more apparent during the

40

1950s and early 1960s. The major drawbacks stemmed from the lack of analytic orientation and ability of many faculties. This led to a number of deficits. First, the academic community in health administration was, in large part, unable to engage in research which could advance the knowledge base for the field in general and for academic training programs specifically. Second, student selection was aimed at young practitioners and failed to attract good students who had no work experience. Because he lacked the traditional academic skills, the practitioner-teacher tended to find his own standing in the university limited in status and promotional potential. There resulted a lack of involvement with university and academic matters in general. Perhaps the one exception was the school of public health, which was largely a federal invention aimed at financing what was conceived to be the needed training in specific public health disciplines. Because the school of public health was a creation of the practitioner-teacher (who at the time of creation wore the hat of the federal bureaucrat), the school of public health became an environment in which the practitioner-teacher could receive promotions, salary increases, and other academic rewards. The result, however, was a so-called professional school whose quality of teaching was near the bottom, if not at the bottom, of the university's endeavors. This fact was tacitly accepted by the faculties, who responded by attempting to produce complete curricula within the school of public health so that the student would never have to leave the school and would never have to face more rigorous courses, tougher faculty, and tougher competition from fellow students elsewhere in the university. Schools of public health, therefore, tended to become isolated islands (of mediocrity at best) within the university. The university in general paid little attention to them, because with vast financial support from the federal government, the school cost the university very little.

Hospital administration programs found themselves in somewhat different circumstances, because they were located in sundry parts of universities, including business schools, graduate schools, schools of public health, and schools of

41

medicine. They too, however, demonstrated many of the same characteristics as did schools of public health. They tended to go their own ways, to isolate their students, and to insulate their faculty from the general academic community in the university. This state of affairs was not happily endorsed. Health administration faculties wanted to be bona fide citizens of the academic world.

As a result, and largely to garner academic respectability, doctoral programs were developed. This achieved legitimacy in two ways. First, the very fact that a doctoral program was offered was one signal to the rest of the academic community. Second, graduates from such programs could be brought on board as faculty members, and thus health administration programs could boast x number of Ph.D.'s, D.B.A.'s, and Dr.P.H.'s. To a large extent this strategy has succeeded. Graduates of these various programs have received doctorates, have become faculty people, have received promotions, and in some cases have moved from the teaching ranks into the ranks of school and university administration.

The penalty, however, has been that the academician has tended to lose touch with the field in which most of his students will practice. His research has tended to be either simplistic survey work or a preoccupation with statistical methodology. For the most part it has been of very little value to the field of practice. Further, some of the doctoral programs in health administration, unlike those in the more traditional academic disciplines, lack rigor, and this leads to a real problem. Assuming that health administration is a profession, and using other professions as a model, we find that other professional doctorates relate more directly to the subject matter which is later practiced. Lawyers receive a J.D. in law, physicians an M.D. in medicine. In both cases the nature, scope, and dimensions of the subject matter are known. Curricula relate closely to the field of practice.

In health administration, however, some of the doctoral programs boast that their subject matter is not confined to health administration but, in fact, is based in economics, sociology, psychology, industrial engineering, and other fields. Are we, in fact, saying that there is no academic disci-

42

pline called health administration worthy of a doctorate? The professor-physician and the practicing physician, or the professor-lawyer and the practicing lawyer, have the same degree, yet the practicing health administrator is apt to have a master's degree while the faculty member has a doctoral degree, and often one in some other field. I recognize that this question is not original with me, but I feel that it has not been examined systematically, either by the field of practice or by education in health administration. It should be.

Lest the accusation be made that this presentation is totally one-sided and critical, I do hasten to acknowledge that the efforts in educating faculty have improved teaching and research. These efforts have produced a generation of educators who are doing a vastly better job of teaching at the graduate level. The new educators, in turn, are attracting better undergraduates into professional programs. The movement is clearly in the right direction and has some definite results to show. The need remains, however, for a rigorous examination of how teachers and scholars are prepared. The first generation model does work, but it probably can be greatly improved, and if not, that should also be demonstrated only after thorough study.

Finally, another measure of success is that health administration programs have, in large measure, gained academic legitimacy. They are able to attract faculty interest from other parts of the university. Their own faculties are receiving joint appointments in other departments and schools. In fact, so much attention has been focused within the university that little time and energy remains for attention to the field of practice, in other words, to the marketplace.

The Marketplace

What is this marketplace of which I have said so much? I will attempt to describe my perception of the marketplace as viewed by the academician, by the graduate student, and by the practitioner. It would be impossible to state all possible disclaimers in advance, and the limits of one point of view will become all too apparent. Nevertheless, I feel there is some

43

validity in the viewpoints to be expressed, even though they may be overstated and incomplete.

The view the academician is apt to take tends to be global and is the result of standing back from the action and looking at it in what is seen to be its entirety. This is completely appropriate. Given this vantage point, academicians wax eloquent concerning the complexities of the field. They pronounce that great changes are abroad in the land; they talk of the new skills and talents required by health administrators, not only to cope with change but more importantly to mold it. They speak of computer technology, of quantitative measures, of the necessity of understanding stochastic processes on the one hand and the social behavior of individuals and groups on the other. They disdain dealing with current problems in the field, and favor the more futuristic approach on the grounds that graduates will learn current practices in the field and that graduates will not be ready to assume major responsibilities until several years after graduation,—by which time the field will have assumed the shape predicted by the faculty in the first place. As a teaching strategy this approach makes eminent good sense. Describing current practices is futile because they will be obsolete by the time the student gets around to trying them out. Furthermore, teaching and research must attempt to push back the frontiers of ignorance and increase our knowledge. Thus the global and somewhat futuristic view of the marketplace is appropriate for the academician. He is perhaps the only one who is able to take that point of view.

The student probably has quite a different view of the marketplace. He may share the faculty's point of view to some degree, but he has another viewpoint, and that involves his place in the market. From his point of view, the market probably consists of job opportunities in a variety of institutions or agencies. The graduate looks at this bewildering array and wonders just what kinds of jobs there are out there, and which one is the best one for him. Should he begin working in a hospital? Usually this would mean a position as an administrative assistant, perhaps in institutional planning or in administrative charge of certain of the hospital's service de-

44

partments. Should he limit his thinking to acute hospitals, to long-term care facilities, to mental health facilities, or to the academic medical center? How many and what kinds of jobs are there in these various institutions? Who can really tell him? On the other hand, should he search for initial employment in the prepayment or insurance business? What kinds of jobs does the Blue Cross plan have for him? What kinds of jobs does an insurance company have, if any? The field is also full of administrative agencies. Most obvious are those in government, primarily at the federal level but also at the state level. These involve traditional public health departments or, more recently, rate-setting agencies, certificate of need agencies, or other planning programs. Trade associations have become more and more visible in the last few years, and these too offer positions for the graduate. But what positions? And what is he expected to do in them? The student has been trained or educated by a future-oriented or globally-oriented academic program. Yet he is expected by his employer to operate in a facility or program which is treating today's patients, or which is inundated with today's paperwork, or in a company paying yesterday's bills today. The field often fails to understand the type of education which the graduate has received. It wonders why the graduate is not as skilled as he might be in today's problems, and the field is not particularly patient with the feeling sometimes exhibited by the graduate that today's problems are not all that important anyway and that the real issues lie some place in the future. So the graduate can be somewhat frustrated when he enters this marketplace.

To my knowledge, no assessment has been made of the marketplace as it relates to the jobs available for new graduates. What should the student's expectations be, and what should be the limitations on those expectations? What direct contacts do the teaching programs have with the marketplace and how accurately are they able to describe it to their soon-to-be graduates?

If the field appears to the academician to be susceptible to computer technology or sophisticated quantitative policy making, if it looks to the new graduate like a bewildering array of jobs of unknown content, to those actually practicing in the field it looks like a maze; a maze consisting of regulations imposed by increasingly hostile units of government, of demands by organized consumer groups, of rapidly burgeoning medical technology and the resulting demand by physicians for that technology, and of promises of full services by government and by prepayment and insurance companies. Finally, of course, the fact of rapidly rising costs and the increasing resistance of the public and private sectors to paying those costs, is the pivot on which the field turns. More and more, the health care administrator's job is involved in dealing with regulations stemming from Medicare and from Public Law 92–603 and other legislation. Huge numbers of regulations emanate from those laws. Furthermore, retroactive application of charity regulations in the Hill-Burton law, state rate-regulating agencies and planning agencies, certificate of need agencies, inspections by the Joint Commission on Accreditation of Hospitals, and validation surveys by the Social Security Administration preoccupy administrators, whether, as institution administrators, they are on the receiving end of this regulatory machinery or whether, as government officials, they are charged with the responsibility of writing and enforcing the regulations. To the provider, all regulations appear to be aimed at reducing payments to him. The practicing field, then, is wondering how, with increasingly limited financial resources, it can produce and deliver the services that are being promised.

As the new graduate is thrown into this field, it often appears to the field that the graduate wants one of two jobs. He wants to become an administrative person in a major teaching center, or he wants to become a policy analyst, if not a creator of national health policy. The graduate finds the policy analyst career more glamorous, while the practitioner needs someone to help him survive in a world of policy and regulation which has already been created.

There are, then, at least three distinct views or perceptions of the field. The fact that these three views contain so many differences does create gaps, lack of understanding, and I suspect, some frustration, for practitioners, teachers, and students. There is a great need to close these gaps, or at least to improve the understanding of all parties.

Having raised a number of questions and described varying perceptions of the field, it is perhaps only fair that this paper should attempt to take a position, if only to serve as a basis for discussion or debate. Admittedly, prognosticating is risky business but there are data, primarily of an historic nature, which can be used to make some judgments concerning the direction in which the field of health administration is headed. In my opinion, the overriding factor is the fact that if there is one point of agreement between the public and private sectors, between business and labor, between provider and purchaser, it is that there are finite resources which can be spent for personal health services. A growing proportion of GNP going to health care will not and cannot last forever. Therefore, practitioners know that their major problem may be to deliver care with what will be limited resources. This is apt to mean the rationing of care in some manner or other. If rationing is in the future, serious questions arise concerning who will be the rationer. Will it be the provider or the government? It should probably be government, but more than likely it will be the provider, because the politician cannot *unpromise*—he can only blame the provider. Second, on what basis will rationing take place? Will it be economic, providing care for those who can pay and denying care for those who cannot? Will it be by age? Will it be by diagnosis, or some other measure or measures? These questions are impending and will become acute issues in the years to come. Meanwhile, the most pressing immediate need, and the preoccupation of most providers of care, is financial survival. More and more financial resources are being controlled. Regulations are being applied to how funds can be used and in what amounts. As regulations become more and more complex, the ability of the financial managers of an institution to deal with them will, in large measure, determine the financial future—and the survival or demise—of the institution.

Regulations will not decrease; they will only increase in number and in complexity. This fact produces two results. Regulation complicates the administrative process, and prob-

47

ably makes it a good deal more expensive for both provider and government; it also means that there is more opportunity for the provider or the recipient of the regulation to play games with the regulations. It is often misunderstood but certainly true that the more complicated the regulation, the tougher it is to administer and to enforce. There exist today people who are expert in gaming Medicare regulations in order to produce maximum reimbursement. As regulation grows, so do the games.

What all this means for the educator is that the student must not be insulated from the administrative realities of regulation and legislation. It is not enough that he or she understand congressional intent or the abstract reasoning behind a hospitals classification system such as that contained in the Talmadge legislation. The student must also be sensitive to the realities of administering an institution or agency regulated by diverse and sometimes conflicting rules. Administrators earn their salaries by making decisions. They make these decisions within an environment, and that environment has become political with a capital *P*. Unless that is understood by the graduate, he or she is at a great disadvantage. Politicians pay very little attention to stochastic statistics and a whale of a lot of attention to counting votes. Graduates emerging from programs this year must understand the legislative process; they must understand the regulatory process at the federal level, to say nothing of the state, which provides the environment in which they will be working for their entire professional lives.

So far, I have been somewhat critical of the educational programs and have, perhaps, placed impossible demands on them. In the limited period of time which they spend in pursuit of a degree, students cannot be expected to learn everything. It is possible to argue that the master's program has done its job well if it recruits good students and graduates them into the field of practice with a working knowledge of the field's vocabulary and some of its major issues, and with a set of values and attitudes which will have utility in the field. Perhaps the field of practice itself should carry on the educational activity from that point forward. It is true that the field does not do a good job in educating the young graduate in his first years. Speaking only of the hospital field, the only one of which I know something, I believe that the typical hospital administrator (if such exists) feels quite distant from the academic community. Most hospital administrators who preside over major institutions to which students or young graduates are apt to be attracted are in their middle 40s or older, and the model of the graduate program they have in mind is 20 or more years old. They tend to feel that the teacher-practitioner model is still the basis of the program, or if it is not that it should be; they tend to assume that students have had pretty thorough grounding in departmental operations and other detailed, practical subject matter. They are apt to feel that the curriculum is still descriptive rather than analytic. Given this frame of mind, they are bound to have a difficult time dealing with the continuing education needs of the young graduate as he enters the field and for the first few years thereafter. Furthermore, the administrator feels that he is paid for administering a hospital, not for educating young people.

The field needs help from the educator in designing programs for the development of young graduates. These programs, however, must be based on joint endeavors; they must not spring solely from the heads of academicians. Practitioners should have a voice too—especially the younger ones who are apt to perceive their own needs best. Perhaps the first fact to be understood by the practitioner is that the field does have a responsibility. It cannot merely transfer its obligation to the American Hospital Association, or to the American College of Hospital Administrators, or to university academic departments, or to the W. K. Kellogg Foundation. The institutions and agencies themselves must help develop means of developing their young people.

Summary

The purpose of this paper has been to identify needs which have not yet been met by health administration education. It is my belief that a great need exists, because the educator does not pay enough attention to, nor understand thoroughly, the field for which he is educating students. This fact causes certain problems or difficulties. The first is perhaps the most disabling of all, and that is one of perception. The academician, for example, tends sometimes to look condescendingly on the field and on its practitioners, criticizing them and their lack of skills but at the same time remaining aloof from direct involvement. On the other hand, the practitioner must recognize the unique and indispensable service which the academician can render. Further, the practitioner must recognize that the field itself shares responsibility for the education of young people.

A second problem, which results from the lack of market orientation or lack of attention to the market, lies in the type of research being produced, or not produced. For example, hospitals have been classified into groups for the purpose of reimbursement under Section 223 of Public Law 92-603. Another classification system has been worked out in the draft of the current legislation sponsored by Senator Talmadge, which purports to reform Medicare and Medicaid. This classification system, too, will be used as a key tool in determining how much hospitals will be paid. Although this classification work is statistical and based on analysis of data (precisely the skills with which the academician is presumably most at home), to my knowledge, none of this work has been produced by faculties in health administration. It should have been.

Although other problems could be illustrated, if I have not made the point by now, I never will. In short, bridges between the universities and the field are needed. My exhortation to the academician is to begin building the bridges. Right or wrong, at this point the practitioner is too preoccupied with survival—in the face of regulation and government controls—to build the bridges that are needed.

Comment

J. Albin Yokie: Since the founding of this country and, for that matter, even before the country was created, we have placed full confidence in education to solve our problems and to meet our social needs. We as a people have firmly believed that education is the key to resolving societal concerns and to meeting individual needs. After 200 years of such faith, it is apparent that education is not, and never can be, the panacea for these matters. In truth, education, at any level or in any area, has its limits and limitations. Recognizing that such limitations do exist can give us a better perspective in approaching education for health administration.

Is health administration truly a profession? Perhaps, at best, one could say it is only an emerging profession. Nevertheless, given the limitations of education and the evolving health profession roles, formalized education in health administration is a necessity and can make a significant contribution to the quality of health care in the United States.

Lawrence Hill makes two valid points in his discussion. I agree that there is a lack of what he calls "market orientation" and a need for better definition of demand for graduates in this field. I also agree that there is a need for greater production of scholars and teachers in the field.

One significant advantage of the academician in the area of health care administration is that because he is not involved in day-to-day health care administration, he has the ability to view the field on a "global" or overall basis and thus to help each of us get a better picture of the totality of health administration. If he is to fulfill his responsibility, he must also deal with future developments and be future-oriented. Thus, he can assist us in stretching our minds and in looking beyond the day-to-day concerns, so that we may grow and be able to deal more effectively with change.

Unfortunately, this very quality which we seek in the academician tends to insulate him from the real world of health administration. Further, because he is dealing directly with students who are entering the field, he has a profound impact on their orientation and values. All too often, the result is an isolation of the student from the concerns and problems faced by health administrators.

An additional factor which sets health administration apart from other professions is the high degree of regulation at various governmental levels. The degree and scope of such regulation in health care is not found in most other professions. While all of us cherish the hope that health care will someday become less regulated, none of us really expects this to happen in our lifetime. In all probability, health care will remain heavily regulated. It will remain so because society will demand it. This degree of governmental regulation must be dealt with effectively in any health administration curriculum or program. Not only must the student be given some basic skills and understanding of the governmental process, but in order to survive he must also probably be given some skills in what sociologists call *patterned evasion*. In short, he must be given some tools to assist him in coping effectively with this aspect of health administration.

My suggestions would be to develop opportunities for greater participation by practitioners in developing and evaluating health care administration curricula, and to provide more opportunities for faculty to interact in an actual administrative environment.

First, I would suggest that practitioners be appointed to faculty advisory committees and that the selection of these practitioners not be limited to graduates of the programs for which they serve as advisers. It would be in the best interests of all to have on the advisory committee a mix of program graduates and non-graduates, all of whom are practicing administrators.

Second, it would seem worthwhile to encourage the establishment of faculty "sabbaticals in administration" wherein the faculty could, for varying periods of time, be relieved of formal teaching responsibilities and actually interact in current health care administration environments. To my way of thinking, this should not be a mere observer function but should involve participative interaction in actual administration strategies and functions. Both the organization in which the faculty member performed and the faculty member himself could benefit from such interaction.

Third, because of the variety of functions in health administration, it is essential that practicum experiences be maintained and perhaps even expanded, on both the graduate and undergraduate levels. Greater attention must be focused on the need to find effective means to bridge the distance between theory and practice. A practicum or administrator-in-training program (AIT) does enrich the formal curriculum. In their report in Volume II of *Education for Health Administration*, on the role of the health services administrator and its implications for education, Allison, Dowling, and Munson cite from their interviews with practicing administrators, that experience has been the best teacher.

A residual effect of such a practicum or AIT program is the stimulation of formal curricula and programs. This administrative experience can provide another opportunity for a joint endeavor of academicians and practitioners in designing health administration education programs.

It is obvious that continuing education will play a significant role in the future lives of health administrators. Greater interaction between practitioners and academicians could improve the quality and content of continuing education programs. It can make the lifelong learning opportunities even more valuable to the administrator.

From my perspective, it appears likely that all the professions will, sometime in the future, require continuing certification of professional competency. We will not be certified as health care administrators in perpetuity but will have to prove our competency periodically through examination, licensure, certification, or some other means. Society will demand such continuing certification. When this does occur, it will reinforce the need for greater interaction between academia and the profession. One of the universities which I attended has as its motto: "Science With Practice." The future development of education for health administration could be best served by adopting that as a goal.

Discussion

Again, the discussion focused quickly on research, with the example of a systems technology for hospitals developed by university-based research and described as still a "Model-T technology" but offering at least the promise of a 10 to 15 percent improvement in hospital productivity. The system has been largely ignored by government and by the voluntary sector. It has been accepted by a commercial enterprise that is now selling it to the field, with some acceptance among professional administrators but with almost uniform resistance from boards of trustees, who have been unwilling to tolerate the disruptive effects of the changes that would accompany its application. "We still don't understand the problem," the discussant concluded.

Some considered that the experience was not all negative. The bridge between research and practice exists, it was suggested, and an example demonstrated research that had proved useful in practice. "You're halfway there," Mr. Hill commented. Others saw the gap as still formidable. A program director said he had proposed a "practice sabbatical" for educators but had not been able to find any practicing health administrators who were interested in pursuing the idea. Another director pointed out that there are two educational models, the graduate school and the professional school. "The professional school must have a profession," he said, "and the profession must have a body of knowledge, which we don't have yet. But without the graduate school approach we never will have it. This won't come without research."

Another suggestion for narrowing the gap was the use of government agencies as training sites. "But we have to have some money to pay the trainees," said a public health physician. "We get some trainees for medicine and public health, but we can't get any for health administration, and the budget won't let me take any students from the schools. So traineeships are drying up. Who is going to pay?"

Again, it was observed that as costs of service go up, more money is required to pay for services and "fringes" have to be omitted. Thus education, research, and planning have the same problem: underfunding.

Barbara K. Knudson, Ph.D. (presiding): The comments here relate to something that underlies the whole of higher education, as well as the whole of this specific part of the field. The need is for some articulation between the field and research and education in the ivory tower sense. We have a unique opportunity here as we search for something which I think is an amalgam of the graduate model and the professional model, and I hope it may be possible to take something from each and to find an approach that will have the best of both worlds. As we seek a solution for the traineeship problem that has been mentioned, I think we would find it if we really believed that the traineeship is an integral part of a person's education. If, in fact, a student can afford to be a student, he can affort to be a trainee. It may seem to require some different resources, but it ought to be considered fully, wholly, and totally a part of the educational process, with the same resources, not different ones. We at the universities generally don't consider the traineeship as part of the educational process. We think of it as some other kind of thing—as a practical experience kind of thing—and that is at the heart of the question that was raised first—the gap between research and the utilization of research. It exists in this field and in all other fields.

The discussion ended with a reassuring comment that the gap between practitioners and academicians may not be as bad in health administration as it is in some other fields. A business school representative observed:

You have a higher proportion of scholarly practitioners and practical scholars floating around in health administration than we have in business administration, and possibly more than there are in law. In business administration the practitioner has been stripped of all his prestige. We have barrels of information about managers—about their stupidity, blindness, lack of tolerance for ambiguity, rigidity, recklessness, and the unintended consequences of their decisions. No wonder they have a hard time listening to professors of management telling them how to do it better! We have completely discredited the practitioner of business administration. I'm saying this because there is enough commerce between research in health administration and business administration that you might catch the same disease. The question is, what systematic knowledge exists about the practitioner's ability to produce intended consequences? Because administrators do get things done. They do produce intended consequences. We don't know very much about that, and in order to understand it we have to study perception. You have to look at the world from the practitioner's point of view, and you have to start with the assumption that he's not an idiot, and he's not a kid, and that our job as academics is not to be condescending; it's not our job to impregnate the practitioner with our brilliance. No longer is the academic's job the collection and analysis of facts about organizational realities which it is the practitioner's job to learn and use as tools. The question now becomes, what can we understand about the perceptual world of the action-taker, what does the organization seem to be to him or her, and how is it that he or she gets anything done? And then, from that research, to develop educational strategies which simply reinforce this incredible human skill that we're all born with to get things done in complex social situations—which reinforce those skills earlier in life, so that you don't realize it only after you've got all your scars. There is a volume of knowledge about this. People have been there before, and have tried to understand how it is that the human mind is conscious of anything. The research strategy is an exciting direction, to try to get around the problem of chronic alienation between the world of research and theory on the one hand and practice on the other.

56

V

Baccalaureate Education in
Health Care Administration

Harold J. Cohen: The "modern" baccalaureate movement in health care administration education began between 1965 and 1970, when a handful of programs was established primarily to train students for entry-level administrative positions in the health care field.[1] An apparently limitless demand for health care administrators in a flourishing economy, the easy availability of federal funding for innovative projects, and a pervasive boom mentality on most college campuses spurred the formation of the first baccalaureate programs.[2] Unfortunately, during this formative half-decade, the baccalaureate programs developed in a vacuum, isolated from one another and from the long-established graduate programs. Administrators and faculty in the latter were bemused by the phenomenon, if they gave it any thought at all. Added to the natural feeling of superiority often displayed by graduate educators toward efforts on the undergraduate level, was a condescension engendered by the 20-year head start enjoyed by the graduate programs and by the fact that many of the first baccalaureate programs were started by small colleges, whose local or regional reputations could not match those of the nationally known universities in which most of the graduate programs were located. In turn, representatives of the earliest baccalaureate programs probably breathed a sigh of relief at not being forced to display their wares so soon to their more experienced graduate program colleagues. Unfortunately, this mutual decision to ignore one another created strong barriers to civilized communication, barriers which today still hamper efforts to establish a closer working relationship between graduate and baccalaureate programs.

The period 1970–75 witnessed a remarkable expansion in baccalaureate programs. Dr. Sue M. Gordon has identified 52 operational programs. Graph V–1 shows the number of

GRAPH V–1

Number of Baccalaureate Programs
By Year of First Graduates[3]

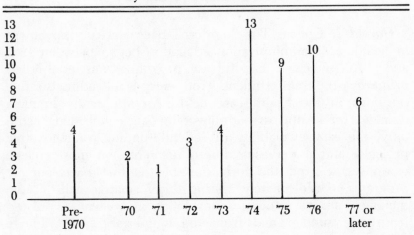

baccalaureate programs by the year of graduation of their first class. Baccalaureate program directors still receive at least two or three letters a month from educational institutions interested in entering the arena, indicating that the movement has not yet crested. *Mirabile dictu,* even some universities with graduate programs in health care administration have established baccalaureate programs. Truly, baccalaureate education in health care administration has become a force to be reckoned with, a sleeping giant whose potential is not yet fully understood. This development has not come without serious conflict. In the early 1970s, with the economy beginning its downward slide, the drying up of government funds for education, and the sudden glut of neophyte administrators for hospitals, graduate programs began to take their baccalaureate counterparts very seriously as competitors

58

for scarce educational resources. Internecine warfare broke out within the organizational confines of the Association of University Programs in Health Administration as some baccalaureate programs sought recognition, membership, and parity with graduate programs. Behavior on both sides was often far from exemplary. Passions eventually cooled and sanity returned, at least partially, if for no other reason than there were too many baccalaureate programs to ignore.

Today, baccalaureate and graduate programs stand together at a watershed. They can continue to coexist peacefully, if unproductively, or they can begin an era of good feeling and cooperation which will be to their benefit and in the best interests of the health care industry at large. Closer cooperation among programs on the two levels depends to a great degree on a better understanding of their respective objectives, curriculum content, graduates, and problems. A discussion of these aspects of the graduate level is beyond the scope of this paper; however, considerable data are now available concerning the baccalaureate level, as a result of Dr. Gordon's study.

Objectives of the Baccalaureate Programs

For several years, some observers have criticized the baccalaureate programs individually, and as part of a movement, for allegedly failing to define their educational objectives clearly.[4] Such criticism usually makes odious comparisons to the crispness with which the graduate programs have presumably stated their objectives and proceeded to fulfill their missions. Are the goals and objectives of the baccalaureate programs really so diffuse or obscure, or are the observers merely uncomfortable with the moderate diversity of objectives which presently characterizes the baccalaureate level? For a field that pays so much lip service to the shibboleth that in pluralism there is strength, we normally cannot wait to standardize and, if possible, fossilize any new development.

In truth, a review of the catalogues of the 52 operational baccalaureate programs reveals a remarkable degree of consistency.[5] Of that number, 42 state they are preparing students for entry-level or middle-management positions, with 34 of these mentioning specific or suggested job titles within distinct areas of the health care field. Sixteen programs also stress their role in preparing students for graduate study in health care administration. Apparently, most baccalaureate programs are attempting to produce administrative personnel for intermediate levels in the hospital hierarchy, an area long neglected by the graduate programs, and for top-level positions in those sectors of the health care delivery system that have consistently been considered unattractive by graduates of the master's programs. Furthermore, a significant number of the programs appear to realize that for the immediate future many of their alumni will have to go on to graduate school to gain entry to the loftier levels of the health care delivery system.

While the majority of baccalaureate programs espouse these objectives, honest and healthy philosophical differences exist concerning the most appropriate raison d'être for baccalaureate education in health care administration. At one end of the spectrum are those who believe a baccalaureate education and experience will eventually be enough to qualify a young man or woman for the position of chief executive of the average community general hospital. Naturally, this view has more adherents on the baccalaureate level than elsewhere. At the other end of the spectrum would fall the belief that because of their traditional ability to produce large numbers of graduates relatively inexpensively, baccalaureate programs hold, or should hold, a natural monopoly in areas such as long-term care administration, which are currently characterized by a scarcity of qualified administrative personnel. According to supporters of this view, the baccalaureate programs should concentrate on these special institutions and not intrude upon the territory of the graduate programs. Strangely, many proponents of the baccalaureate programs, and those who wish to limit their development, can comfortably share this view.

The Baccalaureate Curriculum

Critics and supporters of the baccalaureate movement often argue about the need for standardizing the curricula of undergraduate programs.[6] Critics compare the homogeneity of the graduate programs with the alleged "catch as catch can" attitude of the baccalaureate programs. While I believe representatives of the graduate programs place too much emphasis on the virtues of standardization, many baccalaureate directors have, unfortunately, responded too defensively to legitimate suggestions concerning the possible creation of a common-core curriculum for all four-year programs. The Association of University Programs in Health Administration's Undergraduate Task Force, which I chair, hopes to focus attention on this issue during the coming year by developing a core curriculum which can be recommended to all baccalaureate programs. A review of some of the courses now *required* by the 52 baccalaureate programs included in Dr. Gordon's study indicates that the Undergraduate Task Force may indeed be able to make a significant contribution to the future development of a quality baccalaureate movement by concentrating on this fundamental issue. Table V-1 shows how many programs mandate one or more hours of a particular subject and how many do not require any course work in a specified subject area.

Although Table V-1 is not intended to describe the curriculum of individual baccalaureate programs, it does indicate that some programs may have serious curricular weaknesses. Obviously, anyone should be dismayed to find that 12 programs do not require even one course identifiable as an introduction to the health care field. The low priority given to the political milieu by the vast majority of programs appears to run counter to good sense and to the recommendations of the Commission on Education for Health Administration. Other omissions may perturb those of you with special interest in other areas of a possible core curriculum.

However, there is also cause for optimism. The administration and faculty of some of the baccalaureate programs obviously oppose the concept of a more standardized curriculum because they cannot realistically judge its effect upon their programs. Without real evidence, they fear that they may not have the resources or flexibility to meet the demands of a universally accepted core curriculum. The realization that many of the programs already require a number of courses which might appropriately become part of a future core curriculum should help overcome much of the negative attitude toward reform.

TABLE V-1

Number of Baccalaureate Programs
Requiring Specified Number of Hours of Course Work
in a Particular Subject Area[7]

	0 Hours	1-3 Hours	4-6 Hours	7-9 Hours	10 Hours
Introduction to the Health Care Field	12	19	17	3	1
Political Science and Governmental Relations	38	8	4	1	1
Economics	14	10	13	9	5
Health Law	16	27	6	3	0
Administrative Theory	10	9	17	12	4
Personnel Administration	19	13	13	7	0
Financial Management	7	6	10	11	18
Public Health Administration	42	6	4	0	0
Health Planning	32	9	8	2	0
Medical Sociology	37	12	2	1	0
Quantitative Methods	16	16	12	5	3
Systems Analysis	22	18	9	3	0
Research Methodology	39	10	3	0	0
Management of Specific Health Care Facilities	10	20	6	10	6

Graduates of the Baccalaureate Programs

At least 1,000 students have already completed baccalaureate programs in health care administration.[8] Approaching its silver anniversary, Georgia State University has produced 350 administrators on the baccalaureate level; Pennsylvania State University now has 200 graduates, and Ithaca College is fast approaching the 150 mark. Unfortunately, we know very little about the typical graduate. While Dr. Marshall Raffel of Pennsylvania State University[9] and Dr. Gordon[10] have undertaken in-house investigations of some of their own

62

alumni, no one has yet completed a study covering graduates of all the programs. Shockingly, elementary questions remain unanswered. Who is the average baccalaureate-level trained administrator? Where is he working? What is he doing, and how well did his academic training prepare him for his current position? Will he be ready to assume more responsibility without further education?

In mid-1973, the Bureau of Health Resources Development funded Dr. Gordon's study specifically to answer such questions. Unfortunately, in the spring of 1976, just when the number of baccalaureate-level–trained administrators approached a critical mass and the number of new and proposed programs reached unprecedented heights, the federal government, being unable to untangle its own regulations governing longitudinal studies, canceled the contract for the project. Failure to gather such information will cause irreparable damage to the development of a rational manpower program for health care administration. The directors and faculty of graduate and baccalaureate programs should urge the federal government or private organizations to resurrect quickly Dr. Gordon's study, or to begin a similar project under new auspices.

Major Problems Facing the Baccalaureate Programs: Faculty Quality and Cooperation with the Graduate Programs

Two of the most important problems affecting the quality of baccalaureate programs are the size and competence of their faculty and the need to articulate more closely with graduate-level programs. In her study, Dr. Gordon noted that joint appointments and the use of part-time faculty members from elsewhere within the college or university often made it difficult for the baccalaureate program director to determine how large his academic staff really was.[11] However, Table V–2 clearly demonstrates that most baccalaureate programs have fewer faculty than do graduate programs.

Although there is little data on the experiential and academic qualifications of the baccalaureate programs faculty, at least one observer has labeled a number of baccalaureate programs marginal in view of the small number of teachers

63

holding doctoral degrees.[13] While the baccalaureate programs may indeed have fewer faculty with Ph.D.'s, many baccalaureate program directors and outside observers would dispute whether this truly indicates less commitment to quality. In some cases, the programs' lack of funds necessitated the employment of faculty without doctoral degrees. However, other programs deliberately chose former practitioners as

TABLE V-2

Frequency Distribution of Full-Time Faculty Associated
with Baccalaureate and Graduate Programs[12]

Number of Faculty	Baccalaureate Programs		Graduate Programs*	
	Number	Cumulative Percent	Number	Cumulative Percent
1	6	24.0	4	9.0
2	6	48.0	4	18.0
3	8	80.0	5	30.0
4	4	96.0	8	48.0
5	1	100.0	5	59.0
6			4	68.0
7			2	73.0
8			3	80.0
9			2	84.0
10			4	93.0
11			1	95.0
12				
13				
14				
15				
16				
17			1	98.0
18			1	100.1
	25	100	44	

Source: *Education for Health Administration*, Vol. II, Ann Arbor, Health Administration Press, 1975, p. 99.

faculty. These programs honestly believed that faculty with recent, high-level experience in the health care field would be more effective than faculty with doctoral degrees for preparing entry-level or middle managers. By incorporating more people with experience into their faculties, the baccalaureate programs are merely retracing the steps of the early master's programs, revitalizing an idea which may have been abandoned prematurely at the graduate level. In fact, the inclusion of practitioners may be an important step toward realizing the Commission's goal of establishing more links between academia and the field of practice.[14] In truth, programs on both levels would benefit from a better mixture of academicians and former practitioners; the present high percentage of holders of doctoral degrees on graduate program faculties should probably not be considered an infallible criterion of quality.

Lack of money or deliberate policy decisions do not themselves totally explain the smaller percentage of Ph.D.'s in baccalaureate programs. Both the graduate programs preparing new faculty and the baccalaureate programs will have to change their attitudes toward one another before we see an influx of academically qualified faculty in the baccalaureate programs. Doctoral programs now stress research as the path to success in the academic world. Baccalaureate programs, however, emphasize teaching; single-mindedness about the production of research does not necessarily lead to tenure and promotion. Given the number of new faculty positions on the baccalaureate level, the doctoral programs would be wise to reduce their bias toward the preparation of researchers and to stress the opportunities available to their graduates at the baccalaureate level. In turn, baccalaureate programs must begin to make provision for new faculty interested in research. Today many baccalaureate programs do not have a tradition of granting release time for research. Also, the relatively heavy teaching loads of many baccalaureate programs often do not allow faculty to undertake meaningful research. These conditions must be changed if baccalaureate programs are to attract more faculty with doctoral degrees. In general, however, research probably will never, and should never, become a predominant feature of the baccalaureate programs.

When discussing the quality of health care administration education on both levels, many critics have commented upon the inadequacy or irrelevance of the current curriculum. They all suggest different changes, but most share one trait—they want to add something to the already groaning curriculum. If, for example, you take your sermon from the "Book of Bellin," you discover that doctors do not respect administrators because the education of the latter is not nearly as rigorous as the physician's. The answer, according to Bellin, is to expose the apprentice administrator to a mind-bending basic training in the clinical sciences, creating a crypto-physician.[15] The members of the Commission, on the other hand, find that the graduate programs concentrate too exclusively on institutional management courses, leaving the administrator defenseless in dealing with problems that originate outside the hospital or nursing home.[16] Their answer: more grounding for the student in the behavioral sciences, community and social organization, and the political process, producing what we, as undergraduates, used to call somewhat sardonically the "Renaissance man."[17] The Commission also recommends the expansion of field work and bemoans the fact that some programs have done away with the residency.[18] How is one supposed to cram everything that is allegedly needed into the current curriculum? Since there is little likelihood that more than the traditional two years will be devoted to training administrators on the graduate level, one conjures up an image of the harassed graduate program director trying to meet all the demands made on him by jamming more natural and social sciences into his educational suitcase, only to have administrative theory and data processing pop out the other side.

Might not the answer to the current time-crunch lie in closer cooperation between selected segments of the baccalaureate and graduate levels? Can we really afford to wait until graduate school to expose students to *basic* courses in the social sciences and management? Can we in good conscience devote 3 or 6 or 12 months of a 2-year graduate program to a field placement? I believe we cannot, and I would recommend that steps be taken immediately to rationalize the current system by more closely integrating some baccalaureate and graduate programs. One possible method would be to establish regional affiliations or alliances between selected graduate and baccalaureate programs. For example, Ithaca College and one of the several graduate programs in New England or the Middle Atlantic States should begin to explore possible areas of cooperation. Given the natural barriers to such affiliations, the first steps in this direction would have to be cautious and of a non-threatening nature. For example, faculty members with expertise in the same subject area might begin to meet periodically to discuss changes in their field. Next, joint faculty development seminars might be arranged, reducing the cost of such events for both schools. Then, once or twice a year, faculty at each of the schools might be invited to lecture at the other. Finally, the spirit of cooperation could move into the areas of sabbatical leave and joint use of resources. For example, a baccalaureate faculty member with a master's degree might welcome the opportunity to work with and learn from, a graduate program faculty member with a doctoral degree. Conversely, the graduate-level instructor might enjoy getting away temporarily from the pressure-cooker atmosphere of the university to work with students at a totally different level of sophistication and experience. Exposure to the relatively heavy teaching loads on the baccalaureate level may help him sharpen his own teaching skills and, if nothing else, may make him appreciate the time he has for research at his own university.

After taking these first timid steps, perhaps the affiliates would find the courage to move on to more imaginative and radical cooperative ventures. For example, the two schools could design criteria for choosing a select number of highly qualified students for admission to the baccalaureate program. The graduate affiliate would guarantee acceptance into its program of all the special students who successfully completed the baccalaureate program. At the same time, both schools would have to integrate their curricula more closely. For example, many of the basic management courses now being taught on the graduate level could be left to the baccalaureate program, while the graduate school could begin to concentrate on teaching these subjects in depth or on designing sophisticated independent study projects for these advanced students.

This proposed affiliation would benefit everyone involved. The university program would gain a significant measure of control over the preparation of some of its future students from the day they first enter college. The program would be assured that at least some students would come prepared to pursue truly advanced work, instead of undertaking basic study masquerading under high course numbers as graduate-level education. There would be no need to teach a former history major about balance sheets and the difference between Medicare and Medicaid. Profiting from their relationship with prestigious universities, schools like Ithaca College would be able to recruit better-qualified students. The student would benefit from not duplicating major portions of his costly undergraduate and graduate education—thus avoiding what Dr. Bellin has called (perhaps too severely) a "tedious rehash."[19] The health care industry at large would gain by having new entrants who have had a really high level educational experience which prepares them to meet the challenges of today's extremely complex health care system.

Obviously, the nay-sayers will dismiss this proposal as impractical. They will point to the failure of many similar experiments in the past. They will question the desirability of articulating graduate and baccalaureate programs, even within the same institution. They will say no college or university can submerge its institutional ego sufficiently to circumvent the philosophical and logistical problems involved in such an effort. However, one must recognize much of this seemingly practical advice for what it is—cant which is designed to justify the comfortable decision to do business as usual in the face of an impending crisis.

I recognize, however, that not all colleges and universities may be willing or able to become involved in such affiliations, nor should every student follow this track in participating institutions. Students must always be free to enter graduate programs with backgrounds different from the one I propose. Nevertheless, more articulation between programs is vital and I believe critics of my approach have an obligation to suggest practical alternatives. Talk about closer cooperation between the two levels must be followed by action, or there may soon be nothing to talk about. Both levels must cooperate to protect their own interests and to justify their existence. The residue of hard feeling from the past must be set aside; bruised egos must be soothed and constructive criticism must replace gratuitous sniping. Neither level has a monopoly on virtue or expertise, and both must realize no turf is inviolable. The baccalaureate programs are not marginal. They are new and they have the vitality and adventurous spirit of youth; but they are often inexperienced and could benefit from a helping hand generously extended by true friends on the graduate level. The graduate programs are not becoming obsolete, as some claim. They are mature and knowledgeable, and they have suffered much trauma in bringing health care administration to its present high state. They could demonstrate their maturity by sharing their wisdom and experience with the baccalaureate programs to help them avoid similar pitfalls.

We health care administration educators must soon begin working together in order to avoid the fate of *Tyrannasaurus rex*, cut down at the peak of his power because his pea-sized brain could not bring his strength into play quickly enough to avoid extinction.

Comment

David B. Starkweather, Dr.P.H.: The general assessment of the distance between graduate and undergraduate programs is accurate; however, I would put more emphasis on the confusion over goals, and less on the stress that has been created by competition for resources and arguments over job markets. Without a clear definition of purpose at both, the graduate and undergraduate levels, it is hard to make any sensible determination of where there are complementarities and where there are duplications and voids. I question whether the observers of undergraduate developments are "uncomfortable with the diversity of goals that currently characterizes the baccalaureate programs," as has been stated, as much as they are concerned that the goals are often varied and vague because they have not been developed thoughtfully and realistically. I also suggest that there is not the homogeneity of goals and activities at the graduate level that has been described, but rather that at the graduate level there is a trend toward heterogeneity. I sense that both graduate and baccalaureate programs are now entering a period of sober reassessment of purposes, for the reasons that were defined by Dr. Austin.

Concerning jobs and administrative roles in the field, the fact that 1,000 undergraduates have disappeared into the health administration woodwork without anyone's knowing what they're doing is curious and revealing. It is too bad that Sue Gordon's study has been canceled. But I think that if there were some clarity in the field as to how to use baccalaureate graduates, we would know more—even though we don't have the statistics. I am referring here to the void in the educational developments of the last few years between practitioners and academics. Universities have dumped their educational product into the institutional market without market testing, without market preparation, and then we are surprised that we know so little about what undergraduates are doing, much less should do. I'm not arguing for a simple equation of educational supply matching market demands. That can be misleading. I am suggesting that the arena of articulation between graduate and undergraduate faculties be expanded to include a third party—professionals; and that the important graduate-undergraduate articulation Mr. Cohen calls for be aided, if not mediated, by this interested third party. And perhaps there can be a strange reversal here, where the thoughtful practitioners can mediate a dialectic between academics.

Mr. Cohen commented on the groaning curriculum and what to do about it at the graduate and undergraduate levels. His major proposal is that there be a deliberate integration of graduate and undergraduate education. Specifically, he has suggested that some undergraduate and graduate programs should be integrated through regional alliances. He is careful to say that not all programs should be integrated, at either level, and that not all students should be expected to follow this coordinated track. Without speaking against the alliance, I think there are some major rubs in the proposal for this integration. One rub is for the undergraduate programs, which would have to fashion two curricula that were markedly and basically different: one for the continuing student, with emphasis on the basic sciences and liberal arts and the underpinning breadth of disciplines for graduate professional education; and the other for the terminal student, which would emphasize vocational skills. This would be very difficult for the small faculty, and Table V-2 shows that one-third of the baccalaureate faculties consist of one person.

It is also a rub for the student, who would have to decide very early which pathway to choose—at a time in life when it is difficult to make such decisions and in the face of very limited knowledge about a field and an employment market which is uncertain and likely to change. It is also a rub for the graduate program, which would have two cohorts of students; course work designed for the uninitiated is viewed by others, as Mr. Cohen has said, as tedious rehash.

This is one of those problems that seems to call for an all-or-nothing solution: either abandon undergraduate specialization in health administration, or link all undergraduate education to graduate education in a manner perhaps analogous to premedical and medical education. The former is not plausible, and the latter could lead to the production of preprofessionalized administrators—a meritocracy of managers skilled in the techniques of administration but not knowing for what they are administering—a world of regulators and regulatees who agreed a long time ago that regulation is at best an inevitable evil and that we might as well go along with it.

This brings me to what I think is the key challenge in baccalaureate program development; to develop curricula that retain strong elements of social and biological

71

sciences, humanities, and other liberal arts, while also providing an orientation and application of these to health —i.e., to use health and health administration as the integrator of these studies rather than as a substitute for them. I think that this is possible. I know that it is extremely difficult, and my fears that this is not happening are borne out by Table V-1; 14 programs have 0 hours in economics, 18 programs have 10 hours in financial management of disease factories, and 37 programs have no hours in medical sociology but numerous hours in facility management. I am also worried that the large proportion of baccalaureate faculty drawn from the ranks of administrative practice will lead away from the kind of foundation curriculum that I think is important, or at least to the lack of a mix of practitioners and academics.

As the alliance that Mr. Cohen proposes evolves (with, I hope, the participation of the third party which I have suggested), the trick will be to avoid some natural tendencies, such as: the tendency for employing administrators to put skills and tools for running health factories above an understanding of the human condition; the tendency for graduate faculties to put a higher premium on journal accounting than on the social accountability of professionals and managers; the tendency for baccalaureate faculties to substitute a description of the health industry territory for a broadly based and well-constructed education for civil service—in the best sense of the word.

To respond to the charge that we are dealing, at least in part, with baby steps, I focus at this juncture on undergraduate curriculum developments within AUPHA, which has gone to considerable organizational strain to create the forum for this development. I suggest that the efforts to develop curriculum guidelines be preceded by broad circulation of a statement of the assumptions on which the curriculum and course recommendations for undergraduate programs are based—assumptions about roles, career pathways, and administrative needs of the field—and that the design of curriculum and course suggestions should proceed only after this set of assumptions has received broad comment and at least some effort at consensus. This circulation should be among thoughtful administrators, *public policyniks*, clinician-administrators, and gurus like George Bugbee and Andy Pattullo. It might also be submitted to some students. This would promote the definition of goals and administrative roles that I have mentioned, and would provide the basis for the next stage of educational articulation that seems pending.

Peter B. Vaill, D.B.A.: I sense that there is a general disaffection in colleges and universities these days with new programs. There is not the mood for innovation and new program development that characterized the field 10 or 15 years ago, so any new curricular thrust is up against a generally more skeptical climate, and the null hypothesis is that it's not worth doing.

A second observation comes out of a question; in what sense is a Bachelor of Arts in hospital administration going to be educated rather than trained? Health institutions are, in some ways, the carriers of some of the most cherished values in western civilization including: the commitment to, belief in, and enchantment with, science and technology; the value of life; and the opportunity to pursue happiness. And, it is chiefly through health institutions that the federal government actualizes the injunction of the Constitution to promote the general welfare. They are a class of institutions within which arise some of the most mind-boggling ethical questions that have ever faced mankind, in which the whole post-industrial trend toward professions and the knowledge-oriented society is present in spades, in which minorities and women are finding more opportunities for challenging work and meaningful lives than they find in other institutions, and, finally, in which the ethos of efficiency presents itself in a much more complex fashion that it would in a General Motors assembly line.

None of these values can be understood, much less

73

critically evaluated, by a person who is only trained, not educated. I worry about the possibility of creating an undergraduate experience which efficiently transmits technique and method but which fails to educate the student in the complexity and multifacetedness of these values that I've listed. In my opinion it would be to the long-term detriment not only of the health field but of society if we filled the pipeline with technocrats. I would say all of what I have just said about Bachelor of Business Administration programs also. What I see instead, if we are going to have baccalaureate programs which have something to do with the health field, is an opportunity to create a new kind of liberal arts curriculum. I haven't any idea what it is, but I have an idea that as long as we are talking about a class of institutions in which the traditional concerns of the liberal arts are woven through and through, and about an educational world in which the liberal arts are on the defensive, maybe the opportunity exists to define something called liberal arts for this field of professional practice that would in no sense replace or preempt what we're now doing at the graduate level, but which might form a truly exciting foundation for the more specialized and technical work at the graduate level.

In thinking about what the curriculum for an undergraduate program might be like, I came up with a quotation from a professor at the Harvard Business School who was talking about the needs of the manager of the future. He thought that "the manager of the future needs to understand the nature of himself, the nature of science, and the nature of society, as they relate to the nature of organization." From that kind of Olympian observation some curricular ideas could be developed to form the fundamental content of an undergraduate program in health administration. I would plead with those who feel that a baccalaureate program in health administration is appropriate that they not set their sights on the existence of a market and on the fact that hospital laundries, dietaries, and financial offices are not yet filled with good managers, and that they not simply create programs to fill those needs, but rather that they think of the four-year experience as still a liberalizing experience oriented to a future professional career in health administration.

Discussion

William H. McBeath, M.D. (presiding): I'm reminded of the man who staggered home late at night, tripped over the umbrella stand, and woke up the house. The lights came on and found him sprawled there on the hallway floor, where he looked up at his irate spouse and said, "I've decided to dispense with my prepared remarks and take questions from the floor." We're ready to hear from you.

The discussion emphasized first that what the graduate schools and the field are seeking from the undergraduate program is not a core curriculum but rather a consensus on the scope and level of exposure represented by the undergraduate degree, so that there will be some basis for understanding—in the graduate programs and in the market. The most distressing characteristic of under-graduate education in health administration today, it was suggested, is the confusion of institutional and faculty ambitions with the real needs in the field. The confu-sion is sometimes exacerbated by practitioners who have created the impression that developing an undergraduate program is inexpensive and uncomplicated, and that it can be built around the contributed services of practicing administrators—without a major commitment by the university. In effect, students are misled by the same con-fusion and often seek advice later about where they stand and what their opportunities really are. There is indeed a need for some kind of statement concerning the mission of the undergraduate programs. In the opinion of one participant, the mission should be oriented toward a sig-nificant unmet need for education in the management of

75

functional specialties within large-scale organizations; it was felt that this might be compatible with the liberal arts objectives outlined by Dr. Vaill. When it was suggested that specialization might focus on the *type* of institution (as opposed to a function within the institution), the concept that there are "simple jobs in small institutions and complicated jobs in large institutions" was described as "one of the myths of the field." In fact, administration in large institutions is "insulated by breadth and depth," whereas in the 25-bed hospital or nursing home, and in the small public health department, the institution is very much affected by everything the administrator does.

Another discussant expressed concern that the health administration field had become circumscribed and somehow separated from other human services. Integration of the services of health institutions and other institutions is rare, it was pointed out, and yet most families have more than one problem and need the services of more than one institution. But the curricula in health administration education rarely include anything concerning inter-organizational relationships, which may be one of the most important areas of knowledge yet to be developed: "Health administration programs make less and less sense as time goes on, and what we really need in this country are human services administration programs."

The discussion of undergraduate education in health administration has been going on for years, a representative of one of the undergraduate programs commented,

> It always follows the same pattern. There's always something wrong with the undergraduate programs. The negative approach: They ought to do this, they ought to do that. This is what's wrong with undergraduate education. Yet I suggest there must be something good about them, in view of: their expansion; the support that society has given them through government, state, and foundation funds; and their attractiveness to students. What's good? Why are these programs burgeoning? What needs are they meet-

ing? What human needs are they meeting—other than middle-management competence?

In reply, Mr. Cohen said,

The good news, and the reason for the expansion of the undergraduate programs, is that they fill a real need today when, for better or worse, the total concept of a liberal arts education leaves you with no job in sight. The programs are very practical, and a number of people are coming into them because it is much more desirable to be a health administration major than to be a sociology major or a history major, or what have you. Maybe that's not at the same level as talking about western civilization, but that's very practical to the young men and women who come into our programs. As to why the universities do it, I suppose it's for the same reason they do it at the graduate level; there seems to be a need for it among the students. We are a very profitable part of the college scene now, and I believe this is why the number of undergraduate programs has grown, and this is why they have flourished. There might be a lot of fancier reasons, but this is what it comes down to, and I don't see any reason to apologize for it.

Notes

[1] In 1925 Marquette University began the first formal academic program in hospital administration. The program, which included an undergraduate unit, ceased functioning in 1929. Georgia State University began its baccalaureate program in 1952. Additional baccalaureate programs did not come into existence until the late 1960s.

[2] In 1968 Ithaca College became the first college or university to receive federal support for a baccalaureate program in health care administration.

[3] Sue M. Gordon, "Profile of Baccalaureate Programs in Health Administration," prepared for the Second Undergraduate Faculty Institute, Chicago, May 1976.

[4] Gary L. Filerman, "Issues in Program Development," *Proceedings of the First Undergraduate Faculty Institute*, April 1975, p. 29.

[5] Sue M. Gordon, "Relevance to What? Health Programs in Search of a Goal," presented at the Directors' Workshop, Health Resources Administration, Bethesda, Maryland, August 1975.

[6] Marshall W. Raffel, "Issues in Baccalaureate Program Development," *Proceedings of the First Undergraduate Faculty Institute*, April 1975, pp. 44-45.

[7] Sue M. Gordon, Report prepared for the Bureau of Health Resources Development under Contract # 1-MB-4166, Bureau of Health Resources Development, Health Resources Administration, Public Health Service, May 1976.

[8] Ibid.

[9] Raffel, "Issues in Baccalaureate Program Development," pp. 35-51.

[10] Sue M. Gordon, "After Graduation—Some Data and Issues," *Proceedings of the First Undergraduate Faculty Institute*, April 1975, pp. 82-96.

[11] Sue M. Gordon, Report prepared for the Bureau of Health Resources Development.

[12] Sue M. Gordon, "Profile of Baccalaureate Programs in Health Administration."

[13] Robert DeVries, "Reaction to Issues in Program Development," *Proceedings of the First Undergraduate Faculty Institute*, April 1975, p. 56.

[14] *Education for Health Administration*, Vol. I (Ann Arbor: Health Administration Press, 1975), p. 8.

[15] Lowell Bellin, Keynote Address to the *Second Undergraduate Faculty Institute*, May 1976.

[16] *Education for Health Administration*, Vol. I, op. cit., p. 72.

[17] Ibid., p. 74.

[18] Ibid., p. 73.

[19] Lowell Bellin, Keynote Address to the *Second Undergraduate Faculty Institute*.

VI

Improving the Content
of Education for Health Administration

James G. Haughton, M.D. (presiding): As one of the people who buys your product, I have some ideas about what I'd like to buy, and I don't always get it. Education tends to lag behind programs—in every field. That's true in medicine; it's true in nursing. It's very difficult to keep up with the changing times. I'm not an educator, but I would suspect that it's not too easy to change your curricula to keep abreast of the changes taking place in the field of practice. It's easy for people like me to sit back and tell you what you ought to be teaching, without being aware of what problems we create for you when we say these things. But I still think it's important for you to hear them, so you will know what we expect, and at least you can keep somewhere close to what we think we need.

John D. Thompson: Earlier this spring, James A. Hamilton, one of the more brilliant and certainly the most acerbic of the previous generation of educators in hospital administration, drew an interesting analogy concerning the present generation of academicians engaged in educating health services administrators. "They remind me," he remarked, "of the man who went to the Folies Bergère to study the audience." This was oddly, if accidentally, insightful. Any student of the health services scene today must realize that the audience is actively astir, and that the fruit being hurled onto the stage is not raw material for a new Josephine Baker costume, but represents anger and dissatisfaction with the production. Furthermore, the audience is demanding participation in de-

79

cisions about the script selection, casting, and the price of the tickets. This is the "new theater" with a vengeance. The actors are sometimes in the audience, and the audience often takes a turn on the stage.

If there is one characteristic that marks the difference in health services administration between the two generations, it is not the conflict between the physician and the administrator (although, indeed, that has heightened), it is the conflict between both of these providers and the consumer. In the latter group one must include the organized claques of consumer surrogates, the third-party payers, and public controllers. The new curriculum must address these conflicts in both its content and teaching mode. This presentation does not intend to deal with the proposed content in specific terms. The various task forces of the AUPHA, through the active participation of program facilities, have managed the delineation and dissemination of the basic curriculum components derived from other disciplines. It is now considered time to develop our own amalgam of this content, forged in the almost unique milieu of conflict which characterizes our field.

Dr. Dixon, in an early comment on *Education for Health Administration*, stated, ". . . operationally, however, no matter where the health administrator is working, the role appears to be one that is, by definition, full of conflict."[1] Although this statement was primarily concerned with its implications for the education of health services administrators, I maintain that it applies equally to the field of practice and, further, that the educational content must reflect the practice setting. It is always dangerous to define future academic content in light of today's problems, whether viewed as conflicts or not. The only defense I can offer in so broadly describing "new" content is that some of these conflicts have existed in some form or another since the early days of Davis and Bachmeyer at the University of Chicago, while others appear as themes in both the Kellogg and Milbank reports. More specifically, five such areas will be examined. The first three are concerned primarily with conflicts in the field of practice, while the last two attempt to deal with the educational im-

80

plications of the stress within practice. The practice areas to be examined are the administrator-physician conflict, the public control model, and the quality-cost-accessibility conundrum. The educational perspectives selected are the generalist versus specialist tracks in health services administration programs and the involvement of academic programs in the practice field. This list of five facets of role conflict, while not exhaustive, would I fear prove exhausting to the audience, the writer, and the sponsor of this conference if enlarged.

The Administrator-Physician Conflict

Let us first address the conflict between the physician and the administrator in health services delivery. The past history of this discord is as cloudy as it is pervasive. One facet of this broad area was correctly identified by Dr. Dixon. "The principal problem in the (Olson) Commission," he recalled, "was a lot of animus between those who were public health workers—for which you could almost read "physicians" in those times—and those who were not. I have to report," he continued, "that animus 20 years later still exists; people in hospital administration essentially believe that the enemy is the traditional professional in the field of health."[2] There is now some danger that the release of the Kellogg and Milbank reports within one year of each other might preserve this controversy, in spite of the fact that the content of health services administration, within whatever setting it is being taught, is becoming more and more uniform. It is now time to examine all facets of this problem with the irony and detachment they so richly deserve.

Such an examination reveals that the real conflict is between the concepts of the patients' clinical management carried out by physicians, and the institutional or program management carried out by health services administrators. The old conflict between the physician administrator and the steward was essentially due to the fact that the latter was supposed to be unable to understand the clinical management process. The cloak of the physician's professional prerogative

81

covered all aspects of direct patient care. This cover was later extended by those administrators trained in schools of public health who, although not always physicians, were at least exposed to selected medical problems and, therefore, were supposed to be more aware of the factors in clinical management. In the meantime, the decibels of discord between those who managed the care of patients and those who managed the institutions within which that patient care took place steadily rose, amplified by what were regarded as severe ideological differences between two factions of health services administrators, depending on the site of their training.

A great deal of this latter conflict was pure hype. James Hamilton, speaking of the early days of traveling around with Dr. MacEachern to promote the then new field of hospital administration, said, "We would go to this conference or that convention, and Mac and I would agree to stir up the audience by taking opposing sides. Mac would get up and give a presentation maintaining that the patient was the most important consideration in the hospital. The audience would clap when he sat down. Then I'd get up and say, 'I disagree! Money is the most important factor in the hospital, for without money no patients can be provided the kind of treatment they require.' We really got them worked up." The paradox here, I suspect, is that both Jim and Mac began to believe in their own scam. The tragedy was that many others also believed this conflict was real.

In the meantime, hospital administrators trained by both men began to apply many of the principles of modern management to their institutions. Departmental organization was clarified; similar functional tasks were identified; logistic support systems were put in place; modern salary and personnel practices were implemented; exquisite costing systems were designed; and budgets based on departmental costs and revenue permitted the application of newer internal controls based on identified financial responsibility and public accountability. The systems were applied in all areas of the hospital, except to those functions carried out by the medical staff, such as admitting, treating, and discharging patients.

The medical staff still remained the primary resource allocator of the hospital, through its control of the clinical management of individual patients.

In fact, this clinical management model became more complex with the application of high technology which required increased capital and additional support personnel—which resulted in mounting expenses not directly under the control of administration. The medical staff continued to be unconcerned about institutional costs, however well defined by minutes per meal, hours of direct nursing care per day, or cost per pound of laundry. These measurements, as well as the reimbursement unit based on overall cost per patient day, did not mean anything clinically. Until costs or revenue could be expressed in terms consistent with the treatment patients received, the physician could not, even if he wished, determine the effect of his treatment patterns or caseload on the resources expended by the hospital. The administrator was equally unable to assess this effect, since his reference frame continued to be that of functional departmental cost and revenues.

This inability to express runaway institutional costs in terms that were mutually understandable to the two critical managers fostered the distrust of each for the other and (to return to the original analogy) often resulted in physicians' joining the audience in hissing the administrator's performance. An example of the differential treatment that these two providers receive from a governmental control program is that PSROs can disallow the payment of a hospital bill but will not disallow a physician's fee for that same period of treatment.

Furthermore, there are indications that nurses, members of the largest health profession, are beginning to fashion their own clinical models related to, but still separate from, those of medicine. How much of this is due to a redefinition of the role of the nursing profession in health care, and how much of it is due to a reaction against the standard time-based analyses of patient care tasks so characteristic of recent attempts to impose a functional management model on

83

nursing services, is open to conjecture. Aydelotte warned administrators some time ago that the functional approach failed to fit the real concerns of the nursing profession.[3]

The new content in health services administration must address these problems head on. The concern at this time is not whether it can be done; research at Yale and at the University of Ottawa indicate it can.[4] These two efforts are mentioned because they are the ones I am aware of; there are probably other viable approaches to the definition of the hospital's patient care output in terms understandable to both clinicians and administrators. Today, it is important to explore the curriculum implications of these new approaches.

Permit me to elaborate a bit on one such approach so that these implications can be addressed. For each class of clinically meaningful patient groups, a resource consumption pattern is developed on a statistical basis to provide the "product" cost information which forms the basis for that institution's or program's budget development. Budgets are then maintained according to operating centers and programs, but the extension of these expenses into case cost frames allows a mapping of such costs in terms of patient load. Thus the basis for a system of variance analysis, responsibility accounting, and control of operating costs is provided through a system specifically designed for health care delivery settings.

Of course the variability present among individual patients and medical personnel precludes *certainty* predictions, but careful specifications of criteria should make possible predictions of the *statistics* of resource consumption such that both medical and administrative management can be made more effective. This approach relies strictly on specifications of criteria which, from a medical point of view, ought to influence the pattern of resource consumption.

Given the ability to so classify patients, the benefits occur in two distinct ways. From a clinical point of view, the patient management process within patient classes can be monitored through comparison of expected values of resources consumed with actual values, patient-by-patient. Whenever an outlier is detected, that particular record can be examined to ascertain whether the medical management process might have improved, whether the classification system (set of criteria) was not sufficiently sensitive to predict in that case, or whether the parameters of prediction ought to be changed. This last situation would stem, for example, from such conditions as prescribed changes in treatment and advances in therapy. The peer review process so essential to good health therapy care could be made more effective through such a system.

From the administrative point of view, one would have available a set of output measures (patients treated in each class) by virtue of which control could be exercised over resource expenditures. For an acute care institution, for example, each class of patients would be associated with a prediction of expected resources consumed—length of stay; dietetic, laboratory, and radiology services utilized; drug and physical therapy provided; and other important ancillary resources consumed—thus providing a multi-dimensional yardstick against which each patient's charges and costs could be assessed. Through constant review and monitoring of expectation against outcome and through institutional and regional comparisons and performance reviews, the management of these institutions could be based on their performance with respect to patient-by-patient outcome rather than simply on broad budgetary goals related to activities.[5]

I hope you do not interpret the preceding paragraphs as a major prediction that the development of commonly accepted, clinically meaningful, statistically stable, and fiscally relevant diagnostic-related patient groups will resolve the conflict between the clinician (medical or nursing) and the institutional or program manager. I am not anticipating conflict resolution. All I anticipate is sufficient conflict dampening through the use of common products so that a rational health service administration theory can be constructed, tested, and taught. Such a theory, with clinical management as its base, could then begin to derive production functions for each diagnosis-related group and uncover valid costing, pricing, corporate planning, and evaluative strategies for health care institutions which will radically change curriculum content for the future.

The Public Utility Model

The second and third conflict areas in the practice of health services administration, i.e., those of the state public utility model and the cost-quality-accessibility conundrum, are (at least in the area of health services) really different aspects of the same problem. This problem has been stated in various ways by many in the field. Anne Somers simply calls it, "regulation by an accountable public authority,"[6] and Klarman identifies it as, "the need for a higher superseding level of authority to make decisions when the interests of the individual firm or agency diverge from those of the community at large."[7] The curriculum implications of these statements are obvious. First, both the regulators and the regulated will be trained by programs in health services administration if these decisions by a superseding level of authority are to be related to the field; and second, these authorities will be public or quasi-public organizations.

In many of the program settings, health services administration has been an extension of hospital administration. Consequently, much of the present curriculum has been focused on institutional management, not on the public control of those institutions. Planning content has, for example, been primarily devoted to corporate planning in an attempt to achieve the goals and objectives of a single institution. The faculty has too often adopted the posture of apologist for the hospital rather than of critic. This attitude must change substantially, in framing new curriculum offerings, if programs are to prepare administrators for the various control bodies even now in place.

The setting of most of these agencies has resulted in the generation of a new "word fact" in our profession known as *public policy*. When you have been around as long as I have, you become accustomed to these phrases which assume the illusion of reality once a name has been attached to them.

We have been subjected to such "word facts" as *regionalized health services*, which came into popular use in the late 1940s. Then there were the *all-inclusive rate, progressive patient care, reasonable costs*, and *comprehensive health planning*. It is interesting to trace the rise and fall of these concepts, and one can become rather blasé about their effect on health care delivery. To do so, however, would miss their contributions, which were to widen the field through new insights. *Regionalization* made us study health services in other countries; the *all-inclusive rate* stimulated new techniques for analyzing accounts receivable; *progressive patient care* introduced the concept of stochastic systems into health services management; *reasonable costs* led to more sophisticated cost accounting and financial planning; and *comprehensive health planning*, began, at least, to identify the necessity for consumer input. *Public policy* should, at the very minimum, make us conscious that the various levels of government are our partners and that we had better include legal and political content in our new curriculum. *Public policy* is somewhat different from the preceding "word facts" in that, while they were limited to our field, our concern with public policy is shared by other disciplines, including political economy and history.

Let us examine the public utility model a little more closely, even though it is presently mired in boring detail regarding which costs are to be included—either as retrospective allowances or in prospective rate negotiations. Somehow, the more critical points—which payers are to be covered under these laws (other than Medicaid) and the inability of most of them even to consider the cost-quality-accessibility trade-offs —are never mentioned. Make no mistake, there are some fascinating aspects of rate setting alone, once one gets past the inevitable lawsuits, avoids the adjectives "arbitrary" and "capricious," and considers the problem of equitable payment of similar institutions for similar services. One state's experience in nonmaternity costs for a recent year illustrates the complexity of equitable payments for similar services. It is presented here not to answer how it could be done, but to illustrate the kind of problems that must be faced in a new curriculum that addresses factors in governmental cost control (see Table VI-1).

The central problem in this control arena, however, is that the monitoring of the three critical areas of institutional or programmatic health care (cost, quality, and accessibility) is in most parts of the country (New Jersey being one of the notable exceptions) split, sub-split, and spread among a variety of agencies which share only the initials *P.L.* in their enabling legislation. Cost control is the concern of various state agencies under their own legislative mandate, soon to be joined by six other states receiving some financial assistance through Public Law 93-641. Various Social Security amendments delegate a piece of this action to the Social Security Administration and Social Rehabilitation Service. Quality falls under another agency, the Bureau of Quality Assurance, and its decentralized Professional Standards Review Organizations (under Public Law 92-603). Although this legislation superseded Public Law 89-97 in this area, the SSA and SRS are still the agencies whose payment, or lack thereof, implements the findings of P.L. 92-603. Accessibility comes under another bureau under P.L. 93-641 and its coteries of Health Service Areas.

This litany has been reviewed to underline the present confused and confusing status of Anne Somers's simple phrase and to plead that education in these three areas not be trifurcated, but considered as facets of the same problem, none of which can be treated without the others.[8]

Implications for Education in Health Administration

Let us now turn to a somewhat safer, if no less confused, arena and directly examine two aspects of the educational programs which will influence the new curriculum. In examining the educational problems of training both generalists and specialists in health services administration, we (again) find ourselves prisoners of our own history. Many existing programs in health services administration developed from one specialty, that of hospital administration. Others repre-

TABLE VI-1

Connecticut Hospitals
Cost per Nonmaternity Day
Size, Classification, and Setting, 1974

Hospital	Cost Per Nonmaternity Day	Beds	Classification	Setting
1	$202.67	87	UT	U
2	171.76	821	UT	U
3	151.21	301	MT	U
4	149.54	73	C	R
5	146.84	99	C	R
6	145.43	865	MT	U
7	142.36	440	MT	U
8	139.34	77	C	R
9	136.89	606	MT	U
10	135.54	309	T	R
11	134.11	397	MT	U
12	132.86	497	MT	U
13	131.48	185	C	U
14	129.63	375	MT	U
15	129.38	278	T	R
16	128.34	300	T	U
17	126.89	80	C	R
18	124.98	298	T	U
19	124.55	66	C	U
20	121.94	354	MT	U
21	121.58	227	C	U
22	121.24	213	T	U
23	121.14	148	C	R
24	119.64	131	C	U
25	119.27	368	MT	U
26	118.18	300	T	U
27	116.40	80	C	U
28	115.16	235	T	R
29	115.01	77	C	R
30	114.84	167	C	R
31	108.11	367	MT	U
32	106.16	148	C	R
33	105.24	277	T	R
34	100.35	188	C	R
35	95.34	157	C	R

UT = University Teaching
MT = Major Teaching
C = Community
T = Teaching
U = Urban
R = Rural

Source: Connecticut Hospital Association Management Data Exchange

sent new coalitions of a variety of specialty programs ranging from health education to maternal and child health. In both types of settings, and in contrast to other professional education, the progression was from preparation in the specialties to a more general format. Many students, at least in my own university, are interested in a general program, rather than in a major in one of the specialties; in 1975, 21 of 65 graduates elected such a curriculum. The rest of the graduates selected various institutional or programmatic majors. The problem in educating the former group is not their electing several areas rather than one in which to take courses, but identifying the basic skills which should be taught. They do not wish to become institutional administrators, or planners, or HMO managers. It seems at this writing that in addition to the basic core of epidemiology, financial management, and organizational behavior, these generalists are considering courses in evaluation as their most applicable skill area, along with electives in the institutional and programmatic areas. In these latter cases, courses in ambulatory care are frequently selected, as are electives in environmental health. Recent changes in Connecticut's requirements for town and city health officers, which permit nonmedical public health graduates to assume these posts, have frankly stimulated interest among students in the generalist track. It is insightful to reexamine the local health officer's role with the transfer of the traditional "clinical" aspects to a part-time medical adviser. It is too early to predict the success of this approach, or even to project the specific job market for these graduates. It will be interesting to monitor the generalist program over the next five years.

One area of firm agreement between the Kellogg and Milbank reports is in their recommendations that health services administration faculty become involved in practice. The Milbank report suggests that faculty undertake "periodic, if not continuous, formal responsibilities in the operation of community health services which are relevant to, and will be supportive of, their respective fields of academic responsibility."[9] The Kellogg report is a bit less specific, suggesting that faculty and students participate "in community service, technical assistance programs, and the development of new types of health and medical care delivery systems, and in formulating public policy relating to health."[10]

There is little doubt that health services administration is a practice-oriented profession. It is also quite true that this practice is now changing more rapidly than in the previous ten years, so past practice patterns soon become obsolete. Having directed their attention to doctoral education in order to gain academic respectability, today's health services administration faculties have less practical experience than their predecessors.[11] All these conditions contribute to the need for faculty involvement in the practice area.

In spite of these facts, I find the Milbank recommendations incredibly romantic, while the Kellogg statement responds, I feel, more specifically to the optimal role of an educational institution. I use the term "romantic" deliberately, in that when the faculty recommendations are coupled with the section on research in the same report, one gathers an impression that recreates the myth of the availability of a significant number of teacher-researcher-clinicians to staff programs in health services administration, when we all know these individuals are rare indeed.

My main concern with the relationship of the educational program to the practice field is based on two aspects of such involvement, those of selectivity and role definition. As in the expenditure of any resource, allocation of faculty time to specific areas is critical. In selecting faculty activities, I would plead not simply for the relevance of the practice area to curriculum content, but for the careful choice of specific problems within these areas. Such faculty investments must be directed toward the changing aspects of health services, must have as a focused objective the creation of new teaching material and the testing of new concepts, must be based on the research interest of the program, and must involve students. Practice involvement so defined would generate new curriculum content and could assist in the fashioning of new teaching approaches.

I mentioned earlier that the role of health services educators has in the past been that of apologist for, rather than

91

critic of, the health service delivery scene. If the goal of education in health services administration is the "mental competence necessary to understand the present system and to challenge it," then our students need training in challenging.[12] It follows that the educator must design his curriculum in both an informative and critical frame. This is somewhat difficult to accomplish in a practice setting. That, however, is the contribution that involvement in practice can offer if faculty people are one step removed from practice.

To return to the original analogy, the critic is part of the audience. If our new curriculum is to concern itself with the audience and the play, it will be necessary to spend time on the aisle as well as on the stage. We should not be misled into assuming that such an educational approach is without its own problems. There is a real danger that the programs will lose their practice constituencies. No one likes to be challenged. No institutional or program manager will appreciate a critical examination of his performance. The frostiness between the field of practice and academia is already apparent. The placement of students in practice settings for various periods of time is considered an essential component of the curriculum; if students and faculty are frozen out of such experience, education will suffer.

Comment

H. Robert Cathcart: If you want those of us who are concerned with hot tea and the operation of the laundry, and so on, to become involved in the academic world, you probably should set up some sort of structure or orientation for us to be part of your programs. I appear at a couple of these programs each year, and I'm not quite sure how much value that has to the program, or to anyone. It does cause me to stop and think once a year, and perhaps if that's repeated enough times that's of value in itself. I was very much impressed last night by Dr. Austin's paper, and to note the tremendous development in health administration education in the past few years. I had such an exposure 28 years ago when I attended a program sponsored by the Kellogg Foundation at the University of Minnesota. In that 28-year period there's been a gap. I have been involved in health administration activities, and the change during that time has been profound. You've gone a long way; it's become much more complex, and if you expect me to contribute to that, you have a big educational job to do just on me.

If faculty members come to the clinical setting, the hospital, I suppose we who are laboring there also have a responsibility to create a setting for them, to make it a valuable experience. There are a lot of dumb show type jobs we could do, but I don't suppose you want those. On the other hand, I have enough people on my back, enough people trying to correct and do things differently, so that I want to be sure that the persons who have meaningful duties at the hospital are identified with the hospital and its role and mission. Therefore I'm concerned about ad hoc type people. I'm not saying that I'm against it, but I'm saying that it's going to be important that we work together, so that those who are from academia are well identified with the mission and with the role of the institution in which they're working. I think that can be done. But again, I need that type of leadership from you. This is especially true because Professor Thompson said the faculty should strive to be a critic of the hospital, that the hospital needs to be challenged, and I agree. The hospital does need to be challenged, and I welcome that challenge, because when you challenge us we think harder, we react more responsibly, and we do a better job for the communities which, after all, are paying our bills.

One of the speakers suggested that the chief executive officer of the hospital might already be too preoccupied with just staying alive. I'm sure that's true, but it might also be an excuse. I think there are many who feel harassed but who can and will find time to do things that seem to be important for the field of health administration. For example, I feel much more comfortable dealing with medical manpower activities, and I know much more about specialty distribution and the production of physicians—the numbers, when the peak period is going to come for medical manpower—than I do about health care administration. That doesn't mean I couldn't become equally involved in that subject, when appropriate.

Professor Thompson's paper included a discussion of conflict. Having been in hospital administration for 27 years, I certainly recognize that there is conflict. I would point out that, as he said, conflict between the administration and the medical staff is probably going to be a part of the system for as long as we can envision, but I would also point out that there is now a common enemy—those people outside the hospital, third-party payers, regulatory people, government agencies, and so on, that are driving and putting together the medical staffs and the administration of the institutions. Also, there is growing evidence of full-time physicians who are identified more with the management of the hospital. So maybe some of those factors should be examined and watched, because in a way they tend to lessen the conflict.

An earlier comment seemed to me, as a practicing administrator, to be particularly important—that hospitals and health care institutions are carriers of some of the most cherished ideas and values of western civilization. I am pleased that we do recognize these human values, including the value that patients need to be recognized as very important persons. If there is some way that you as educators can help us build into our systems more and more of this recognition of the human and emotional needs of our patients, we as practitioners would be very much pleased. I wish I knew how to advise you to prepare people in that respect. Perhaps you who are educators and know how to motivate people can help us to do this.

William C. Richardson, Ph.D.: Professor Thompson has noted that over the past ten years the AUPHA, through its several curriculum task forces, has been active—and, I believe, quite successful—in delineating the "basic curriculum components derived from other disciplines" which are necessary for graduate-level education in health services administration. Further, considerable progress has been made by graduate programs, of all ages and academic locations, in moving toward balanced curricula that include the basic disciplines relevant to management and which provide opportunities for applying those disciplines to the practice of health administration. Nevertheless, educators find that the complexity of the environment that awaits their graduates is increasing so rapidly that what may have appeared five years ago to be the ideal curriculum design, today forms only a sound basis on which to build.

Professor Thompson aptly notes that the task before us in improving the content of education for health administration is to develop our own amalgam—one that draws on various disciplines and skill areas and which is specifically fitted to health services.

This amalgam requires a sophisticated faculty that is able to bridge the distance between difficult analytic techniques and a rather turbulent array of practice settings. Consider again the implication of what Professor Thompson has described for education. The example was given of an approach to measuring the hospital's patient care output. This approach would permit monitoring the patient management process by comparing expected values of resources consumed with actual values on a patient-by-patient basis. It would also provide administrative control through exception reporting and through analysis that takes account of patient mix, practice style, and so on.

Until quite recently, there has been little interest in, not to mention capability for, formulating patient care appraisal, or program and institutional management, in terms based on clinical management as proposed by Professor Thompson. But a number of familiar factors have perhaps inevitably led to the need for what he calls "the development of commonly accepted, clinically meaningful, statistically stable, and fiscally relevant diagnostic-related patient groups." What I find particularly striking is that these same factors have been responsible

95

for the emergence of regulatory or monitoring agencies at the state and local level, with their respective concerns for cost, quality, and accessibility.

It is not necessary to elaborate on these factors. The increasing emphasis on procedure-oriented medicine in a fee-for-service context, institutional reimbursement on a cost basis, and the public's expectations with regard to the ready availability of secondary and many tertiary services have resulted in a remarkable variation in performance —however measured—and in a per capita cost escalation that is startling to say the least. Also sobering is that over half the cost of all physician services for those under 65 is now carried by health insurance; for hospital services the fraction is over three-quarters. Moreover, for the employed population, over 70 percent of premium dollars is paid by the employer.

The point, of course, is that the pressures for public accountability through regulation have been increased not only by the diminution of the usual market forces, but also by the concentration of dollars paid out by large purchasers in the private sector and, more notably, by government. In short, important elements of the public are in a position to find out what is being received for the dollars expended.

The first area discussed by Professor Thompson, the administrator-physician conflict, has certainly been greatly altered by the requirements for public accountability imposed by external agencies. Whether the inherent conflict will be dampened by the development of a clinically based management approach seems to me not so important as the recognition that the future content of health administration education will have technical aspects with three important attributes: first, they will be specific to health services but widely applicable to a variety of delivery settings; second, these technical aspects will of necessity build on, and apply, a diversity of disciplines and skills; and third, these elements of the curriculum will represent concepts and methods as useful to the staff member of a monitoring or regulatory agency as to the program or institutional manager. Professor Thompson has cited a specific and quite fundamental development that calls for future curriculum elements' possessing these attributes. Other potential developments could be cited in such areas as financial management, service area definition, and assessment of consumer preferences.

The factors that I listed earlier would seem to assure that the requirement for public accountability will not diminish in the future. Not so clear at the present time is the degree to which such efforts will be concentrated at the state level. This obviously depends greatly on the form that national health insurance eventually takes. But I would fully agree with Professor Thompson that health administration education can no longer confine itself to program or institutional management. Nor does it make sense to have isolated programs focused only on training for ambulatory management, health planning, health policy analysis, and so on.

The educational amalgam referred to at the beginning has been characterized as being specific to health services, built on a graduate-level disciplinary and skill base, and as providing a common body of knowledge for practitioners in operating settings, as well as for those in coordinating and regulatory settings. Professor Thompson has demonstrated through his own work at Yale how this body of knowledge can be developed. There are a number of other examples around the country. Cursory observation would suggest, however, that the number of graduate programs in which substantial work of this sort is going on is limited. It would appear that the most successful settings have at least the following characteristics: they work in collaboration with faculty drawn from a variety of schools or departments on the campus; they have a core faculty with disciplinary training but which is primarily interested in solutions to health services problems; the core faculty maintains close working relationships with practice settings of different kinds, and the student body is made up of individuals with a range of

97

career interests. In these settings one observes exactly the kind of investment of faculty time that Professor Thompson prescribes; an investment that yields new curriculum content while providing both faculty and students with the opportunity to test and apply more abstract material in the context of the complex operating setting.

I noted at the beginning that it takes a sophisticated faculty to achieve these ends for current and future students. The available pool of faculty able to combine analytic skills with a sufficient interest in, and familiarity with, the field of practice is inadequate; and the opportunities for existing faculty to strengthen their competencies seem unduly limited. On the other hand, the conditions seem to be present for improving the content of education for health administration in most programs. The opportunities exist for collaboration with field sites; faculty from a number of disciplines show increasing interest in health services; and the academic reward structure in most settings seems to be broadening the notion of research to include the creation of new knowledge through demonstrations and other applications.

In summary, the five areas of conflict examined by Professor Thompson, and particularly the more broadly defined "conflict" between providers and the public, have indeed established a unique milieu. It is one in which adept and sophisticated management is increasingly essential for programmatic or institutional survival, and in which little is taken for granted. The demands on health administration education should be no less rigorous.

Discussion

The discussion began with a suggestion that in addition to the conflicts between administration and medical staff within institutions another, and perhaps more significant, level of conflict may be emerging, resulting from the institutionalization of care and the rising expectation physicians have of administration. The increasing number of physicians on hospital boards of trustees and the questions about the role of physicians in Health Systems Agencies may be evidence of this new kind of conflict. The basic issue is: Who is going to run the show? Educational programs should make plans to prepare for this.

One comment was that the institutionalization of care has had little or nothing to do with where care should be given but rather with controlling the delivery of health services. "We *must* teach our students to live with conflict," said a program director. "They have to be aware that the decisions they make are going to be full of conflict, and they have to know that there are no pat answers." As administrators inevitably become involved in clinical matters, more conflict is certain to result, and the conflict will be useless, wasteful, and destructive unless something is done about the effective education of physicians in administrative concerns. "If the physician can determine how his practice and his decisions affect the hospital, he may become involved, but I'm lucky if I can get them to come in and talk about patient care," said a director. Another observed that the programs have done a good job of training managers as managers but have not communicated with the professionals. And yet the professionals are expected to understand administrative problems and to support administrative decisions. On their side, it was suggested, doctors and nurses want to do things and make decisions that require management expertise, but they want to *be* doctors and nurses.

Another view of the administration–medical staff conflict was expressed by a public health physician who pointed out that although the regulator can be an ally of the administrator in dealing with physicians, the opportunity is ignored. Instead, "the hospitals and hospital associations are fighting all our efforts to regulate costs." The relationship of hospital administration and regulatory authorities follows a well-established pattern, a program director suggested. First, regulation strengthens the state hospital associations. Next, the state associations begin to feel their strength and assert a "Let's take 'em over" attitude. When this doesn't work, a third phrase ensues and can best be described as "We'll sue the bastards." Finally, hope for working out some kind of *modus operandi* begins to emerge.

Professor Thompson was challenged concerning the method of getting physicians to understand the impact of their decisions on hospital operations and costs. In response, he presented figures on cost per nonmaternity day in hospitals according to size, classification, and setting. He stated that costs are "an extremely valuable monitoring tool" for use with physicians and that they have been used effectively. It was agreed generally that health administration education programs are a logical resource for the kind of information that must be presented to physicians, and that this must become a major mission of the programs. It was observed, however, that the difficulty of directing physicians' attention to this kind of information has led to a defeatist attitude.

Dr. Haughton (presiding): Everybody assumes that because an internist is a fine physician, he can run a large department of medicine, or because a surgeon is a fine surgeon, he can run a 500-bed surgical service in a hospital. That's absolute nonsense. Three years ago, recognizing this problem, we talked with the faculty of the health services administration program at the University of Illinois. I asked how we might work out an arrangement in which some of our brightest residents, who someday may become heads of departments, could learn something about health service administration.

We've now developed an affiliation with the University of Illinois, so that any medical resident or family practice resident interested in health system administration can simultaneously pursue a master's degree in administration. The first graduate of this program is now the director of our general medical clinic, and it's the best-run clinic in our entire health center. It serves some 300 patients a day and is extremely well organized, because this young man is not only a fine clinician but also a health services administrator. This suggests another opportunity for health administration programs on campuses where there are university hospitals or teaching hospitals.

I am most interested in health administration education for the resident in clinical training, because it is at that time that he is beginning to be a part of the life of the hospital. While he is in medical school, I doubt that administrative training can have the same impact on his future behavior, because at that time he's not too much involved in the hospital. But as he goes up the ladder in his residency, becoming a junior resident and then a senior resident, he begins to participate in the committees of the hospital and in the management of his department, and at that time this kind of training will have its greatest impact on his future behavior.

Notes

[1] James P. Dixon, "The State of Education for Health Administration: Views from the Kellogg Commission," in *New Directions in Graduate Education for Health Administration* (Chapel Hill: Department of Health Administration, School of Public Health, The University of North Carolina, 1975), p. 105.

[2] Ibid., p. 104.

[3] M. K. Aydelotte and W. R. Hudson, "A Socio-Engineering Problem: The Nursing Profession," *Nursing Outlook* 10, no. 1 (January 1962): pp. 20-23.

[4] R. B. Fetter, J. D. Thompson, and R. Mills, "System for Cost and Reimbursement Control," *Yale Journal of Biology and Medicine*, May 2-3, 1975 at the Continuing Education Program, School of Health Administration, University of Ottawa.

[5] The definition of costs used in this presentation is the same as was proposed in a previous paper, i.e., costs are "hospital expenses (1) specifically classified by a standard chart of accounts; (2) allocated directly or distributed to service departments according to a uniform method of apportionment; and (3) transformed into unit costs by dividing them by consistently defined and generally acceptable units of service." This definition of cost is not without problems. Many economists claim that one cannot cost a single product in a multiproduct firm because of the joint-cost problem. The troublesome aspect of such a position is that it has no utility in solving the problems of managing, planning, or budgeting medical care programs or institutions. Industry has faced this problem by elaborating various cost accounting approaches which approximate product

costs for management. Hospitals began to apply these techniques in attempts to separate inpatient costs from ambulatory care costs in clinics and emergency rooms, where both use the same building and share common ancillary services such as radiology and laboratory. What is now proposed is the extension of this approach into diagnosis-related group costs.

[6] A. R. Somers, *The Philadelphia Medical Commons: Mounting the Guard*, Blue Cross–Blue Shield Publication CA 5401.

[7] H. E. Klarman, "Planning for Facilities," in *Regionalization and Health Policy*, ed. E. Ginsburg, 1976.

[8] Somers, op. cit.

[9] Milbank Memorial Fund Commission for the Study of Higher Education for Public Health, "Final Report," (manuscript) 1975, p. 50.

[10] *Education for Health Administration*, Vol. I (Ann Arbor: Health Administration Press, 1975), p. 6.

[11] J. D. Thompson and G. L. Filerman, "Trends and Developments in Education for Hospital Administration," *Hospital Administration* 12, no. 4 (1967).

[12] S. P. Kramer, "Education for Equality?" *Commonweal* 8, no. 3, p. 8.

VII

New Strategies for Universities in the Education of the Professional

Nathan J. Stark, J.D. (presiding): I have found that the staff of the W. K. Kellogg Foundation really keeps its feet to the fire. In doing so, it finds ways of disseminating information to all of us in this field and, more importantly, it is always around to help us implement the programs the Foundation has funded. We are fortunate that we have been joined here today by the president of the Foundation, Dr. Russell Mawby.

Russell Mawby, Ph.D.: We're delighted that all of you have been able to attend this conference, and we're grateful to those of you who have had a part in the development of plans, to those who have presented the major papers, and to the discussants. But I think the most important impression I have had after joining the group today has been the spirit, the sense of enthusiasm, and the liveliness of the discussions, both formal and informal.

I come from an academic background, from a university faculty, as do many of you, whether from an academic responsibility, or professional practice, or wherever, and we've all been to too many meetings. So our hope is that this is not just another meeting. I think it was the intent of those responsible for developing this program and of each of you in making a decision to be here, among all the alternative uses of your time and energy, that this will not be just another meeting. The whole process of thinking about this important area of the organization and administration of our health care services, and about the educational process by which

103

leadership is prepared for this field, is most significant and timely.

As Nathan Stark has indicated, the Foundation has been involved in this field for a long time. We regard it as an extremely important part of our total program. Those of you who have read Kellogg Foundation literature or who have received what we call "request declines" have often been told that we don't support conferences except as they may relate to an important area of program interest. We are concerned with knowledge utilization. It's our feeling that one of the problems of our society is that we *know* a lot better than we *do* in most fields of human endeavor, and that the real challenge is to mobilize resources in new and more effective ways to serve the needs of people and communities. So it is our hope, as it is yours I'm sure, that this conference will indeed mark a new point of departure.

For many of us the challenge will always be, *so what?* And so we'll be concerned in working with you individually and collectively as you go back to your individual responsibilities in trying to ensure that the kind of dialogue and exciting ideas shared here, and the enthusiasm engendered here, are indeed reflected in action. Our thanks to each of you for being involved in this program and for being part of this group. We look forward to our continued association with you.

Nathan Stark: Higher education in the United States is passing through a period of transition as it seeks to respond to new clienteles and the needs of a rapidly changing society. Within the last eight years we have seen a proliferation of commissions and task forces aimed at resolving problems associated with these new needs. Studies such as those of the Carnegie Commission have identified several relative certainties about higher education in the future. We know that enrollments will not continue to increase dramatically and that the costs of higher education are becoming a larger proportion of our gross national product. We have learned a great deal about the attitudes of faculty and students, and studies have revealed that many graduates will find increasing difficulty in obtaining jobs.

On the other hand, we are uncertain about the future attitudes of the public toward higher education and about the role of higher education in the affective and creative areas of human development; we see evidence of growing polarization of campus constituencies, and we do not know how soon advancing technologies will influence the structure and delivery of higher education. In spite of uncertainties, we must develop policies and strategies for addressing problems that will continue to confront us in the future. Clark Kerr has pointed out seven such problems:

1. Applying the principles of social justice to higher education.
2. Producing the trained manpower the nation needs.
3. Academic reform leading to a consensus about what constitutes a good general education.
4. Resolution of problems related to the governance of universities.
5. A major policy decision about the number and variety of institutions that ought to be available in the next 25 years.
6. The need for mechanisms to make higher education available in the future in external modalities and non-traditional approaches, and to meet continuing education needs.
7. Determination of where the responsibility lies for financing higher education in the future.

We are challenged by the Kellogg Foundation to develop policies and strategies for addressing the problems that will continue to confront us in the future. Having identified a few areas of certainty and uncertainty and having pointed out some national problems related to the future of American universities, I can assure you our speaker's views will be most enlightening. Dr. Harold Enarson has devoted his entire professional life to higher education and government service in an exemplary fashion. In his academic role he has served on the faculties of several universities—in many capacities

105

as an administrator—and he is currently the President of Ohio State University. In his government service Dr. Enarson was an examiner for the Bureau of the Budget, Executive Secretary of the Steel Industry Board, a consultant to the National Securities Resources Board, and a Special Assistant to the White House. He will share with us his views on "New Strategies for Universities in the Education of the Professional."

Harold L. Enarson, Ph.D.: As you can see, I am presently the beneficiary of the twentieth century triumphs of modern scientific medicine.* This plaster cast immobilizes a "non-displaced spiral fracture" of the right fibula, and the crutches provide precarious mobility. The origin of crutches is lost in antiquity, undoubtedly the clever invention of an illiterate carpenter. No priestly professional is likely to have been half as clever with hands and materials. The plaster cast is the loving contribution of professional medicine. In the name of advanced medical science and technology, it imposes a cruel combination of Egyptian mummification, Spanish Inquisition purification through suffering, and Elizabethan disregard of plain cleanliness. A leg mummified in a cast is deprived of air, sunlight, water, soap, and breathing. Granted, it is not a matter of medical record that the feet breathe. But why else does a grown man luxuriate in putting his feet outside the heavy covers on cold winter nights? Why do the "best and brightest" at the Medical Center of Ohio State's College of Medicine affirm by their silence that Harold Enarson's foot and leg do not need to breathe—to feel the sweet breeze, the gentle touch of a soapy washrag, the coolness that comes from blessed escape from confinement?

The Enarson leg is inconsequential. But tens of thousands of legs and arms tortured in casts are not. We are told that the American space program yielded a technological harvest of new materials and technologies. Right now, we, the afflicted, would settle for a desperately needed invention—the lightweight, cool, flexible cast, with zippers. I can imagine the

* Dr. Enarson appeared at the conference with his foot and leg in a plaster cast as the result of a recent injury.

ad: "A Tool of the Ages, for All Ages." The ads would serve as a natural companion to Geritol ads on the Lawrence Welk show, and to ads for ski resorts.

I am deadly serious. Any reasonably proficient engineering student of materials could build a better cast. Why hasn't it been done? Because American medicine and American engineering, while they enjoy space on the same campus and separate-but-equal access to football tickets and parking, are light years apart. They meet, if at all, at the faculty club, where conversation rarely touches on the plight of the wounded of the earth.

But enough of highly critical personal testimonial. For if there is folly in the practice of medicine, there also lurks the wisdom of the ages. Recently, I discovered in the attic of a relative's home in New Mexico a delightful book which provides instant perspective on the state of the medical arts in England and the United States in the 1850s. Spencer Thompson's *Dictionary of Domestic and Household Surgery*, published in 1856, speaks directly to the treatment of fractures. (It also tells me more than I care to know about leeches; they are hazardous when affixed in areas near the nostrils or other apertures of the body.) Thompson writes, "Care must be taken, if the person has been accustomed to much alcoholic stimulant, that it not be *unduly* abstracted, otherwise the powers of the constitution will be so reduced that the reparative process cannot take place, and the fracture will remain un-united."[1] (Italicized in the original.)

I knew it. The six o'clock double martini does double duty, restoring the spirit and in mysterious alchemy knitting together the ravaged ends of bones as well. Oh, ancient wisdom! Oh, modern miracle! One wonders whether even the Chinese barefoot doctors practicing traditional medicine yet possess such insight.

Thompson's dictionary has a page or so on "Physicians." It is nicely tucked between the definitions for "physic" and "pickles." I quote in part:

As long as the education of the physician was so infinitely superior to that of the medical profession at large, the prestige which attached to the title was its just due. It still is its just due

107

as the tribute to the mark of high attainment, but it is not just when paid to the exclusion of the profession generally, the members of which, as a body, whatever their title, must now, or at least in a few years, be all as nearly on a level as the difference between man and man permits. Nay, more, the medical profession, as the education of its members is now conducted, must become the most highly intellectual body of men in the kingdom. The studies of a medical man *must* embrace the widest possible range, from the simplest truths of mathematics and of natural philosophy, to the latest developments of practical psychology, and within this range their knowledge is *real, true* knowledge, the knowledge of the manifestations of God in his works; and their deductions from the knowledge must be the alleviation of the physical and many of the mental evils of fallen man, and higher still, their prevention: *For it must ever be to the honour of the medical men of the present age, that though their bread may be said to be got through the misfortune of their fellow-men, they have been ever the foremost to point out how these misfortunes are to be avoided. They have been the first rousers and the chief leaders of the sanitary movement* everywhere. In large cities, and in the metropolis especially, there always will be, probably in an increasing degree (and it is expedient there should), a division of labour among medical men. One will take the skin, another the eye, another the chest, and so on, as his particular department, and will attain such acquirements in connection with his own department, as will give him an extra claim to confidence when that is concerned. Especially in obscure or difficult cases; but this cannot be with the kingdom at large, and in the provinces, the great mass of disease must continue to be the care of the general practitioners, whose experienced leading members must, under the present system of education, become what the physician has been.

The native eloquence of this passage led me to wonder how nurses were perceived. Again, Thompson is not one to equivocate. He writes, "All bad habits, such as snuffing, smoking, and it, perhaps, must be added, drinking, are insuperable objections; likewise the habit or necessity of making unusual noises, such as humming or habitual cough. Neither should nurses be great talkers: Some patients are much annoyed by the garrulousness of their attendants. A nurse ought to be a light sleeper, awake to the slightest call or movement, and no snorer—a light mover about a room." Thompson had not heard of professional nursing. However, he did say, "Some amount of education is absolutely necessary, especially the ability to read writing. Without it the most serious mistakes may and have occurred." Thompson, even as his counterparts today, was not without compassion for the plight of nurses. He wrote, "A nurse ought to be made to go out in the open air for exercise, for at least an hour in the day."[2]

I stumbled upon another reference to nursing that seemed vaguely relevant. The *London Times* in 1856 described nurses as being "lectured by committees, preached at by Chaplains, scowled on by treasurers and stewards, scolded by matrons, sworn at by surgeons, bullied by dressers, grumbled at and abused by patients, insulted if old and ill-favored, tempted and seduced if young and well-looking."

Today, as we all know, nurses view themselves as independent, highly trained, highly skilled professionals with a unique contribution to make in a diversity of settings. In the words of one director of nursing, "Nurses today are no longer pliant, submissive handmaidens, selfless mother substitutes, who passively carry out orders. Nursing is a *profession*." (Emphasis supplied.)

So is virtually every other occupation, job, or skill in the American economy. It is not enough to work at an honest occupation which meets the needs of the society. The word "professional" is the highest accolade, whether for skiers, basketball players, musicians, or secretaries to congressmen. The term "professional" is juxtaposed with "amateur." Even burglars pride themselves on professional skill. Only in sex and politics is the gifted amateur held in high social esteem.

In the common frenzy for the prestige associated with professionalism, many skills and occupations become professionalized—or try to. Firemen, policemen, social workers, YMCA secretaries, reporters, counselors, artists, executive secretaries—all think of themselves as professionals. And professions spawn subprofessions. The academic world takes all this very seriously and tries to make sensible allocations of tasks between the professional and the subprofessional. The professionals in all fields take the matter even more seriously. And rightly so—after all, jobs are at stake.[3] The "subprofessional" who can pull a tooth invites the wrath of the dental profession and the intercession of government. This example can be duplicated throughout the professions.

We deal here, of course, with word magic, one of the oldest, most enduring ways of establishing status and dominion over others. From earliest times, professionalism has been embraced in order to convert a craft or occupation into a protected monopoly. Biblical literature refers to the soldier, the scholar, the lawyer, the priest, the tax collector, and many others. In the Middle Ages, Chaucer could describe in his *Canterbury Tales* the man of law, the doctor, and the clerk. Always, the professional has been a person of special competence whose service is protected by the power of government.

William McGlothlin distinguishes occupations from professions as follows:

> Professions are intellectual, learned, and practical. They have techniques that can be taught; their members are organized into associations; they are guided by altruism; and they deal with matters of great human urgency. These characteristics allow modern society to legalize monopoly through the licensing of professional people, much as the earlier societies permitted only a sharply restricted number of medicine men. A profession is master of a difficult and extensive body of knowledge over which it has exclusive control. No one can execute the tasks assigned to the profession without this knowledge, and no one can acquire the knowledge without the profession's approval. Only members of a profession can perform its tasks and these tasks are so crucially important that society would suffer painfully if they were not executed, or if they were executed poorly. . . . Society allows a profession to be a monopoly because it is convinced that the profession is dedicated to an ethical, or altruistic, ideal in serving society. The profession's ethics, its code, is at the very heart of its professional practice. A society will find other ways of obtaining services if a profession ignores the fact that its privileges are awarded for so long as it aids and serves but does not exploit its clientele.[4]

110

McGlothlin's definition of the professions is the commonly accepted one. You will find much the same definition set forth in the textbooks. But are we to take such pretensions at face value? I trust not.

We are told that professions are intellectual, learned, and practical. Presumably all others, such as bankers, professors of poultry science, and TV writers, are therefore nonintellectual, nonlearned, impractical. Nice put down. We are told that the professions have techniques that can be taught. Of course! But so do barbers and bricklayers, extension agents and agents of the CIA, among others. We are told that professionals are organized into associations. But so are farmers and fishermen, bricklayers and bankers, and criminals. We are told that the professions are guided by altruism. Let your mind dwell ever so slowly on what this says about the rest of the working population: The Beverly Hills psychiatrist is altruistic; the home nurse in the hills of Kentucky is not. Park Avenue surgeons are altruistic; volunteers in nursing homes are not. Lawyers and dentists and optometrists are altruistic; the many whom they serve are not. Now, really!

We are told that another mark of professionals is that their work is of great social value. But this is hardly a useful distinction. Plumbers and electricians, managers of nuclear power plants, and, yes, politicians, also do work of great social value. We are told that professionals are masters of complex bodies of knowledge requiring long years of intensive preparation. But so are the best of stockbrokers and the best of businessmen. This, too, is hardly a workable distinction. We are told that professions have codes of ethics. Indeed they do. But there is precious little evidence that lawyers and optometrists, for example, operate on a higher ethical plane than do college professors or plumbers. In reality, there is only one test that truly controls. Occupations are transformed into "professions" only when public policy sanctions the public protection of monopoly status. To argue otherwise is to indulge in nostalgia and wistful hope.

It would be nice if the Lord could rattle the universe ever so slightly and let us start all over, banning from our vocabu-

111

laries words that so easily corrupt, so often confuse. For as long as we are mesmerized by words, we shall be incapable of looking with freshness of eye on things and events around us.

Over the centuries idealism has been part of the great heritage of the learned professions. But that legacy has been seriously flawed by shattering events, and everywhere the professions are on the defensive—against the ambitious thrusts of new occupations which want part of the glory and the gravy, against one another (as with the warfare of lawyers and physicians), and above all against the rising tide of public discontent with on-the-job performance.

A growing number of Americans do not see the professions as the professions see themselves. Academic standards are perceived as sophisticated job protectionism. Entrance tests are viewed as clever devices to screen out minorities as well as the unconventional. State bar exams and similar credentialing tests are viewed as high hurdles cleverly rigged to protect the interests of the professions rather than the public. The claim of professional altruism elicits a cynical guffaw from the consumers of professional services. Too many have paid too much for services indifferently delivered.

Nowhere is the rising tide of discontent with traditional professionalism more manifest, more bitter, than in the health professions. The American public is mostly indifferent to the internecine warfare of the health professions. The pleas of the nursing profession for a place in the sun are heard only in the hospital corridors and in the remote reaches of professional journals. Similarly, the rear-guard defenses of physicians who assert the primacy of physicians over all health care everywhere are heard only in the echoing cloisters of AMA convention ballrooms. The struggle for professional status as between physician and nurse is only the most publicized of the border skirmishes which waste the energies of the health professionals. In my view, the American people look with mingled disgust and indifference on all such struggles for role, status, privilege, and pay.

Incantations about the glories of the health professions, along with promises that they are about to be miraculously interdigitated into new patterns of coordinated health care, will not suffice. The foot knows where the shoe pinches; the leg knows where the cast suffocates; and the sick everywhere know from personal experience that hospitals, nursing homes, and clinics fall far short by all tests. Our health care delivery system is neither humane, efficient, nor economical. And a heavier dose of standard edition professionalism is hardly the cure.

I do not pretend to know the answers to American health care, any more than I know the answers to a congested environment and a clogged political process. Plainly more of the same won't do—not more hospitals, not more traditional medical schools, and not more emphasis on technology and modern business management.

One of America's leading businessmen told me recently, and I quote, "We have learned that after a point it does very little good to put more dollars into the system. It's dysfunctional." I do assert that there is one place where the public is entitled to look for solutions. And that is the American university, the home of all the professions. For the best and the worst that our professionals practice is inculcated by the university. If provincialism is nurtured, it is the university that does it. If real teamwork is ever a reality, it will be because the university finally fostered it. If nurses and doctors and ophthalmologists, engineers and management specialists, and students of the political process are ever to learn to work together in shared concern for human health, it is here, in our universities, that we must all surely begin. And if that most elusive of goals, the ethic of concern and conscience, is to be advanced, it is here, in our universities, that the first timorous advances must be made.

The grand design of the professions, long overdue, can begin only with the redesign of the university, and its system of governance. But that is another talk for another occasion.

Still, speculate just for a moment on the easy victories that lie so close at hand, if only our professionals would abandon, ever so briefly, the protection of their academic redoubts, and seek out and engage in conversation their colleagues in other areas of the university. The faculty club could be neu-

113

tral ground, a kind of Noah's Ark where exquisitely specialized academics and practitioners could meet to discover shared interests and matching talents. Doctors might meet lawyers, and engineers might meet both. The danger of contamination is slight, the possible dividends great. In such an effort we might rediscover that zeal for excellence in service to others which alone justifies any claim to recognition and reward.

In the face of sickness and pain, all pretension should be put aside. What does it matter that we have elaborate status hierarchies—professionals, subprofessionals, superprofessionals. All we deal with, really, is the human condition—all of us at some time helping, at some time helped. Oh god of medicine and nursing, why cannot thee invent a cool leg cast, with cooling zipper, air holes, apertures for itching? Of such modest and mundane achievements, heaven on earth is built!

Notes

[1] Spencer Thompson, *A Dictionary of Domestic Medicine and Household Surgery* (Philadelphia: J. B. Lippincott and Co., 1856).

[2] Ibid., p. 372.

[3] Recently, the National Labor Relations Board ruled that newspaper editors and reporters are not "professional employees" within the meaning of the National Labor Relations Act. The Board's majority said that its conclusion does not denigrate journalism as a calling or question in any way the quality of the work product of journalists as a class."

[4] William J. McGlothlin, *The Professional Schools*, (New York: Center for Applied Research in Education, 1964), pp. 4-5.

VIII

Achieving Quality in
Health Administration Education

John Kralewski, Ph.D.: When considering quality in higher
education, one is tempted to evade the complexity of the
issues by simply quoting the Socratic prescription to attract
superior students and to provide intellectually stimulating
and supportive learning environments that draw out their
innate abilities. Unfortunately, in today's tumultuous academic world, with its extreme cost and equality pressures,
neither of these is easily achieved. Even though health administration programs attract good students, they are faced
with a myriad of conflicting contextual forces that in many
ways go beyond those that led John Gardner, when he considered higher education in general, to note his "concern with
the social context in which excellence may survive or be
smothered."[1] Education for the professions must also deal
with difficult content issues in rapidly changing fields of
practice.

Health administration programs are particularly vulnerable
in this regard because they are dealing with an evolving field
not yet clearly defined, and because they must bridge quite
diverse disciplines—e.g., management and the medical sciences—to accomplish the educational goals. Furthermore,
the content peculiar to the health administration discipline
is only beginning to be explicated, based largely on the
empirically derived body of knowledge evolving from the
field. There is agreement that graduate education in health
administration is more than a relevant selection from the
smorgasbord of course work developed for other disciplines,
but there is little agreement on what is unique to the field.

115

Discipline definition is therefore a paramount consideration central to the development of excellence in health administration education. Unlike well-established disciplines, health administration lacks the rigorously defined content and structural characteristics that ordinarily provide identity, support, and continuity for an educational program. The interdisciplinary faculty involved in the program, therefore, often lacks the experiential base necessary for a direct identity with the field. This, of course, does little to clarify the health administration field or to develop the discipline further. Under these circumstances, some programs are unable to develop the critical mass necessary to influence either the field or the academic setting and often gain little respect for their activities. The academic base for health administration education similarly reflects this lack of clarity and adds to the confusion with a growing variety of schools (ranging from allied health to public affairs) spawning graduate programs. Some of these programs have little organizational support and are treated as areas of emphasis consisting of one or two courses rather than as distinct disciplines.

There is evidence that this proliferation of programs is just beginning. Many academic administrators view the health field as one of the few bright spots for the future and are eager to participate in the perceived expanding market for graduates, often with the lowest possible investment. Institutions that are more deliberate in the development of new educational programs all too often find it difficult to withstand the twin pressures of students' wanting access to these gatekeeping health administration programs and the promise of federal funds to underpin their financially troubled organizations. Therefore, although the direction of education in this field is at best unclear, there is unsettling evidence that this rapid expansion, lack of discipline definition, and economic retrenchment in the academy could lead to a serious decrease in quality.

In the past, one might have argued that the marginal role played by the administrator in the health field did not constitute a distinct discipline nor warrant more than an *area-of-emphasis* approach to education. The social responsibility of the administrator in today's health care field, however, and the increased emphasis on this role in the provision of health services, dictate far greater attention to issues of substance and quality in educational programs. This is particularly true if, as the Commission's report suggests, we are to expect the health administrator to assume responsibility for ensuring the accountability of the health care industry to society. In order to fulfill their similar public accountability commitments, academic institutions engaging in health administration education must therefore develop rigorous, high quality educational programs and must do so in the uncertain, rapidly changing environmental settings described above. The environments are further complicated by federal funding policies that often discriminate against some organizational settings, and by state legislators and university administrators who must decide which programs should be supported, what level of support is necessary to sustain a program, and the extent of support feasible for their universities or colleges.

Many of these issues affect higher education in general, and other disciplines have faced similar problems during their formative years. In fact, similar issues—and the inability of individual academic institutions to deal with these problems —precipitated the development of program and school accreditation in the early 1900s. According to Dickey and Harcleroad this accreditation served "to meet the social needs for improved higher education and the individual needs of the better colleges and universities for protection from the competition of unqualified—even dishonest—institutions."[2]

Accreditation in this context evolved from a concern over federal intervention in the quality issues of higher education and the unwillingness of the states to assume responsibility. Educational institutions themselves, with impetus from various professional groups who depended on the educational programs to maintain standards of excellence, forced the accreditation issue. As noted by Miller, the accreditation process thus developed focused on two major areas: "those areas oriented toward society at large or public functions; and those oriented toward institutions and programs of study

117

or educational functions."[3] The public function centers primarily on consumer protection by identifying educational institutions and programs which meet established standards of quality. Educational functions deal with improvement of educational standards and programs through the involvement of faculty in curriculum planning, development, and self-assessment.

In light of these conditions (and as with higher education in general), two major quality goals are paramount in the health administration field: identification of the body of knowledge and skills peculiar and essential to health administration and setting educational standards dealing with this content; and development of learning environments which include the necessary resources to achieve excellence as measured against those standards. Academicians who are teaching and conducting research in this field, practitioners who are applying the resultant skills and knowledge in the work setting, and consumers who ultimately use the services must join in these efforts.

More systematic research is needed to determine the appropriateness of the content, design, and structure of graduate programs, and a forum must be provided for practitioners, academicians, and consumers to address these issues. The AUPHA has done much to provide such a forum and must continue to play a leadership role in exploring curriculum content, coordinating role studies, and developing task forces to help further define the health administration field and graduate education within the field. The task forces on functional areas such as planning and financial management, and on institutional areas such as long-term care, have explored program content and structure. As a result, the task forces have helped keep the educational programs in touch with the rapidly changing field, and have helped develop an identity for health administration. Accreditation must correlate with and underpin these efforts. An effective accreditation process should not be directive nor should it serve to create exclusive domains for professionals. It must, instead, synthesize information from academicians, practitioners, and consumers to establish minimum levels of performance. The Accrediting Commission on Graduate Education in Hospital Administration, using data from the AUPHA studies and other sources, has developed at least beginning standards and has assisted programs in the process of self-assessment. External validation through program accreditation or some similar method of program review is central to this process, since the regional and school accreditations, while good, cannot hope to achieve the in-depth analysis needed at this time to assure quality in this evolving field. Furthermore, program accreditation must be carried out by an agency that has a peer group constituency broad enough to review this multifaceted field objectively and yet focused enough to establish precise standards for the field. There is no basis for conflict between school and program accreditation in this regard, nor is it imperative that both be accomplished through the same organizational structure. Both serve useful purposes and neither should dominate the other. The costs associated with multiple accreditations within a school are of course a great concern and must be minimized through joint accreditation visits. The common element in health administration education, however, is the program of study, not the academic setting; therefore the umbrella organizational structure for accreditation must be program-oriented, if it is to address the quality issues in the many differing academic settings successfully. To increase the effectiveness of accreditation, much more effort must be devoted to acquainting potential students and employers with the quality of the graduate programs. As standards become more clearly identified, they must be widely publicized, and annual reports should clearly specify the degree to which programs meet those standards. The strengthening of accreditation through these mechanisms will assure the integrity of the process and will more fully address the public accountability question.

The second phase of this process, achieving the standards through the development of learning environments, centers on resource development and the development of supportive organizational structures for graduate programs. To establish high quality programs, academic institutions must not only have clearly established standards to work with; they also must have, or develop, the capacity to meet those standards. The academic and organizational location of the program and the university commitment are extremely important factors in achieving these educational goals. The accreditation process and the external validation of a program can only assist in establishing standards and help the institutions assess the degree to which the program meets those standards. Thus accreditation is, first of all, a process that furnishes public protection by identifying programs that meet basic requirements. But it also provides the incentive for academic institutions to establish quality programs, since validation is extremely important to their constituencies. As a result, it helps answer questions of resource allocation at the university level.

In many cases, academic administrators faced with financial crises tend to evade the hard decisions (which programs should continue and which should be terminated) and, instead, simply support all programs at a sub-optimal level. Similarly, pressures to provide a broad range of educational opportunities in every academic setting—in order to increase accessibility and equity—cause academic administrators to pursue this course. Health administration is, of course, only one of many programs caught in this dilemma. At a time when job opportunities in other fields are declining and institutions are seeking new markets for their graduates, health administration looms large as a new field of endeavor. The rush to establish programs in a wide variety of academic institutions is causing state legislators and state commissions on higher education to ask penetrating questions regarding the resources needed to establish such programs. The standards, criteria, and identification provided by professional associations and accrediting agencies are important inputs in this decision-making process and contribute considerably to the quality of the resulting programs.

The question of program location has been discussed at length during the past few years as programs have proliferated and a diverse range of academic institutions have become involved as sponsoring agents. Much of the discussion has centered around program financing. Financing is only one facet of this complex issue, however, and one must address the broader question of the parent organization's commitment to excellence and its ability to develop the critical mass necessary to conduct a quality program. To a degree, health administration programs can develop at a level beyond that normally engaged in by the parent organization, but probably only while outside resources (federal or other) continue to be available. In the long run, programs assume the character of the sponsoring institution, and if that organization is characterized by graduate programs with a 20:1 student-faculty ratio, no research, and little or no structure, the health administration program will eventually be similarly characterized. Specialized accreditation, while not ruling on the appropriateness of a specific organizational setting, must fully apprise institutions of the resources and commitment needed to establish a program and must assist in deciding whether they should do so.

To ignore the financial and organizational difficulties faced by academic institutions in developing accessible, high quality health administration programs would, of course, only justify the protectionist concerns often generated by self-enforced quality control measures and would ultimately lead to a loss of public confidence. Accrediting procedures and other external validation mechanisms must guard against the protectionist approach that led Oliver Wendell Holmes, and many others since, to conclude that the professions are a conspiracy against society. Therefore, efforts to increase quality in health administration education must be accompanied by mechanisms that assist academic institutions in deciding whether to develop health administration programs (that meet the established standards) or to forego that academic area and gain access to programs in other settings.

While programs devote considerable attention to the development of financial resources, they often neglect their most important asset—their faculty. Although faculty development is important in any educational program, the present state of the art in health administration and the unique design of these educational programs make this factor especially important in assuring quality. The rapid expansion in the number and size of programs has brought many new teachers into the field—most of them directly out of Ph.D. programs. Pressures to develop depth in functional areas of the programs have brought many from other disciplines (e.g., financial management), some of whom have little knowledge of the health care field. Similarly, the structure of some graduate programs brings together interdisciplinary faculty from a number of schools within the university to teach courses for the health administration program; these faculty members, while extremely capable in their own disciplines, often come with little understanding of the health administration field or the goals, philosophy, and character of graduate education in health administration. Faculty development is therefore crucial to the development of quality in these graduate programs and must be addressed in a formalized manner. Faculty involvement in accreditation site visits has been very useful, as has the participation of faculty in the AUPHA curriculum task forces. Such vehicles as sabbaticals and professional meetings are useful but much too limited; sabbaticals, for example, occur too infrequently to deal adequately with the problem.

I suggest that programs must go far beyond these efforts and should form consortia (possibly regional) to strengthen their faculty. These endeavors could include: development of intensive peer relationships among schools; faculty exchange on a relatively short-term basis (possibly for a quarter or semester); regional seminars for exchanging research information and for developing collaborative research projects; and programs designed to allow students to apply course work taken in one of the participating schools toward degree programs at their parent schools. The student exchange approach would become increasingly important as programs continued to broaden their concept of health administration, while developing depth in functional areas; this is likely to occur in an era of zero economic growth in the academic setting. Many programs will not have the resources to achieve excellence in all areas of health administration by themselves; therefore they will find it necessary to rely on strengths derived from interprogram relationships or to specialize in one or two functional or institutional areas. Programs will have to devote much more attention to pooling resources among schools within the universities—and, indeed, among universities—in order to develop the critical mass of talent necessary for quality educational programs. Therefore, the Kellogg Commission's recommendation to develop centers of excellence in health administration may best be realized by developing consortia of university programs, each emphasizing an area of excellence and sharing that excellence with the other participants, rather than one autonomous program playing that role for an entire geographic or academic area.

The relationship of a teaching faculty to the field of practice is an important issue in faculty development. Controlled consulting and technical assistance are promising in this regard and should be encouraged. Involvement in the administration of the health science center in the academic milieu also has merit, both in providing exposure to the practical setting and in gaining visibility and identity for the health administration program.

To accumulate sufficient resources to enhance quality while at the same time increasing program accessibility for students in states that lack graduate education in health administration, consideration should be given to the development of integrative mechanisms between states, such as the Western Interstate Commission for Higher Education (WICHE) and the Southern Regional Education Board. These programs were developed primarily to assist students in states which do not have educational programs in the health sciences to gain entrance to the highly competitive programs in other states. In essence, several states allocate financial resources to a program in a neighboring state, thus reserving a certain number of positions for their students. Most agreee that this has helped to strengthen the quality of the parent program or school while assuring the contributing states access to these educational opportunities at a cost far below that of even a marginal effort of their own. In some geographic areas this approach would greatly increase the resources available to a program, would give the program a strong regional role, and would avoid the proliferation of marginal programs. Programs in the more populous areas of the country could modify this approach to integrate resources among colleges or universities within their state systems.

In the final analysis, human and financial resources and contextual support can furnish only the potential for quality in health administration education. The program director's leadership ability and commitment to excellence are vital catalysts in building a quality program. Directors of graduate programs must, therefore, be part of a reference group committed to excellence and must be in a position to influence the organizational unit which sponsors the program. There is a growing concern regarding the quality of the academic administration of our institutions of higher learning and, in response, training seminars are being developed for individuals in those positions. Examples include the programs sponsored by the Association of American Medical Colleges for academic administrators in medical schools. Directors of health administration programs are probably more qualified than most academic administrators. Nevertheless, their leadership skills could be strengthened by more rigorous development of peer group relationships among program directors and by improvement of specific educational administrative skills, e.g., in establishing behavioral objectives, program evaluation, and the development of environments that enhance learning. Leadership is, of course, frustrated unless the program director holds an organizational position that allows him or her to influence the academic institution. Little has been done to explore these relationships, even though there is evidence that the director's role is a major factor in determining the quality of a program. At a minimum, directors must control the resources allocated to the program and, optimally, they should in this context report directly to the chief executive officer of the sponsoring institution. Without this direct line of authority, issues relating to quality, and to other aspects of the program, are subject to negotiations among diverse power groups at the lower levels of the organization. The further delineation of these aspects of graduate programs would contribute greatly toward assuring quality at the levels referred to by Miller as "those many other subtle variables that so greatly contribute to quality in higher education."[4] Leadership in this regard is that all-important ingredient that makes the difference between excellent and creditable but lack-luster programs.

Returning now to one of the initial premises, student selection is unquestionably a very important factor in achieving quality in a graduate program. Unfortunately, we know very little about the selection process, and even less about its outcomes. In an attempt to inject rigor into the "personal insight" selection techniques used by program directors in the past, there is now a rather dramatic shift toward screening examinations, such as the GREs and ATGSBs. Efforts have also been made to expand the pool of applicants and to attract better students to the field. While these activities are extremely worthwhile, they need to be expanded in two major ways. First, intensive research should be initiated dealing with selection criteria and the relationships with performance in the graduate programs and in the field after graduation. Second, I believe that we must develop stronger links with the field of practice as a recruitment mechanism, with at least some of the screening and testing of interests and leadership abilities taking place in the work setting before students are admitted to the graduate programs. I am persuaded by Aristotelian philosophy in this regard endorsing the provision of marketable skills in undergraduate education and a broadening graduate education after experience in the work setting. Close ties with the field would also give programs an opportunity to establish management development programs for their graduates with large health care institutions. These connections would greatly enhance the graduate program's ability to achieve a quality program which extends into practice.

Summary

Much has been written about consumer protection and public interest in higher education, and painful lessons have been learned from experiences with marginal, sometimes fraudulent, educational endeavors in a host of fields. In the past, health administration programs have remained aloof from these problems. The field was characterized by a relatively small number of programs located at very good universities, and the programs were headed by charismatic leaders who, in most cases, were committed to excellence. As a result, health administration enjoyed relative tranquility in the tempestuous milieu of higher education. Today, however, higher education in health administration is facing the same problems and criticism experienced by other fields in the past; our challenge is to build on those past experiences in addressing the present-day quality issues in our field. While the interdisciplinary nature of health administration education and the ambiguity of the discipline bring peculiar problems to the arena, most of the issues faced by these programs today are quite similar to those faced by other higher education programs in the past. In addressing quality issues, most educators focused on curriculum structure and program content, and, to a degree, on the quantity of available resources. Program accreditation evolved as a mechanism to establish standards in these areas and to assure a modicum of consumer protection by assessing program performance according to those standards. The merits of this approach have been demonstrated and documented and must be fully endorsed in health administration. This is particularly true since the curriculum content peculiar to health administration is only beginning to be elaborated, and educational standards are at best embryonic. If, however, we are to fulfill our public interest commitment in this field, we must go beyond these measures. Effort must be devoted to the quality as well as to the quantity of program resources—with immediate attention directed toward faculty development. Programs will undoubtedly find it difficult to carry out this function independently; however, the development of close working relationships between programs seems to hold considerable promise. Larger, well-established programs must assume leadership in this regard and must do so with a collegial rather than an elitist approach to cooperation. Similarly, student selection techniques must be improved, with attention to methods that will balance scholastic achievement with the ability and commitment to apply knowledge skills in a manner consistent with the public accountability role of the health administrator. A closer working relationship with practitioners in selecting and professionalizing students offers some advantages in this regard, but is only one of many approaches that must be explored and carefully evaluated in order to improve the inputs brought to the educational environment by the students.

Attempts to control quality in higher education inevitably lead to limitations on the educational opportunities available to students and, to a degree, act to protect practitioners' jobs. As the number of graduate programs continues to expand and the job market becomes more competitive, pressures from practitioners to limit enrollment will certainly escalate. The public interest is not served by quality assurance mechanisms that unduly restrict access to gatekeeping educational programs, nor by those that can be misused to maintain lucrative job markets for those practicing in the field. Therefore, while greater effort must be devoted to quality issues during this time of rapid expansion in the field, equal effort must be devoted to assuring reasonable access to the programs. Regional arrangements similar to those developed in other higher education programs (WICHE, for example) offer considerable potential in this regard and open other avenues for program support.

Many of the issues addressed in this paper deal with the important question of integration within, and among, educational environments. The nature of health administration education and the resource limitations within academic settings cause the integrative functions to take on a great deal of importance—much more than is normally found in other higher education programs. The role of the program director is, therefore, a critical ingredient, and leadership in this position is essential to the development of high quality programs. The role of the program director is not well defined, however, and lacks uniform academic acceptance and recognition in the many institutions sponsoring graduate education in this field. To help clarify this role and to establish more clearly its identity within academic institutions, a series of studies should be initiated by AUPHA in collaboration with others concerned with health administration education. If the health administrator is to represent the public's interest in the delivery of health services, program directors carry similar public interest responsibilities for creating educational environments that will lead to this end. The further development of this capacity therefore must be considered one of the highest priorities in the field today.

Comment

Frank Moore, Ph.D.: I would like to respond to three themes developed in Dr. Kralewski's paper: first, the quest for identity as a discipline and as a prerequisite to the development of excellence in health administration education; second, the relationship of the accreditation process to program quality; and third, how program location affects program quality. These themes are presented as much in terms of their relationship to survival in the uncertain academic setting as in their direct relationship to the issues of attaining quality in graduate education for health administration.

Health Administration as a Discipline

Medical school and graduate school models, with strong departments organized on disciplinary lines, may indeed lend an air of permanence and stability which interdisciplinary programs do not enjoy. However, any plea for disciplinary discreteness based on the dynamics of formal university organization may run counter to the objective of excellence. The pitfalls are many. Perhaps we can take some lessons from our brethren in the social sciences. Present disciplines in the social sciences are arbitrary composites of content, as Campbell has noted: "Anthropology is a hodgepodge of all novelties that struck the scholarly tourist's eye when venturing into exotic lands—a hodgepodge of skin color, physical stature, agricultural practices, weapons, religious beliefs, kinship

128

systems, language, history, archeology, and paleontology." Likewise, "geography is a hodgepodge of land-surface geology, of industrial development, of innovation diffusion, of social ecology, of political territoriality, of visual perception of aerial photographs, of subjective phenomenology of mental maps."[5]

As these collections of interests emerged as disciplines, they inevitably were organized into decision-making units called *departments*, with the concomitant process which Campbell has termed the "ethnocentrism of disciplines." The effects of this departmentalization are familiar to all observers of organizational behavior in the academic institution:

Communication patterns are affected. Sharing of preprints and reprints, reading of dissertations, and informal shop talk become predominantly intradepartmental. Books and journal subscriptions become limited to one field. Annual reviews, abstracting sources, newsletters, and program notes promote the tendency toward intradepartmental centrality at the expense of extradepartmental, peripheral developments. This departmental grouping of communicators fosters a drift into idiosyncratic language that eventually becomes unintelligible to outsiders. Edmund Leach has noted that such idiosyncrasy may be exaggerated as an ingroup solidarity device: "What is depised as jargon by the out-group becomes the hallmark of quality by the in-group."

These symptoms of tribalism, nationalism, and ingroup partisanship are frequently further reinforced by national organizations of educators and their counterpart practitioner organizations (e.g., Association of Teachers of Preventive Medicine, Association of Teachers of Maternal and Child Health).

Competition becomes the norm at the expense of interdepartmental collaboration. Pressures on the student to master the content deemed central to the department increase, often at the expense of elective options in other departments or schools. Competition for

129

space and other resources intensifies. Competition for good students and their subsequent indoctrination with the departmental philosophy erect further barriers to cross-departmental collaboration.

In brief, the organizational dynamics artificially reinforce the "ethnocentrism of disciplines." This circumstance often leads to definitions of quality and excellence which are predicated on purity, discreteness, and academic elegance, thus addressing the internal quality issues.

As Dr. Kralewski suggests, there is an external or, in his terms, a public accountability, issue which extends beyond the academic setting and which must concern and involve both the faculty and the graduates entering the field. In a field that is currently characterized by interdisciplinary preparation, and where demands in the work setting range across many technical and interpersonal competencies, any drive toward disciplinary discreteness may conflict with the practitioners' definition of quality. Campbell has coined the phrase, "the myth of unidisciplinary competence," and has argued convincingly that competence is a collective product, not embodied in one scholar or discipline. Thus, we must carefully examine these two perspectives of the definition of quality and attempt to achieve a balance between those elements necessary to achieve academic respectability (and thereby compete favorably for institutional resources) and those elements in the practioners' (i.e., public) definition which suggest that inputs are required from multiple disciplines. I am not suggesting that these definitional perspectives are incompatible. On the contrary, the practitioner and the academician can, and often do, achieve a common perspective concerning the end product of the educational process. What I am suggesting is caution. While striving for identity and quality in the internal, academic sense, we must be aware that organizational dynamics may lead us to excesses of disciplinary discreteness and raise barriers to collaboration—which if carried to extremes can decrease the competency of the faculty and thus the quality of the educational process and product. We must be careful not to equate improvement in educational standards with increasing disciplinary discreteness.

Accreditation and Quality

A second major theme is the role which accreditation plays in reference to quality in education for health administration. Again, Dr. Kralewski notes the public function and the educational function as the two principal foci of accreditation. As accrediting bodies and their processes seek to serve these two interests, they must be equally circumspect regarding the two definitional perspectives on quality and excellence. If the established standards of quality used to identify educational programs for the public purpose are solely or primarily derived from faculty self-evaluation, research, and planning, there is an inherent risk that the educators' perspective on quality will be passed on to the public function. The practitioner's contribution in formulating these standards must receive equal weight if adequate balance is to be attained. When these two viewpoints are compatible, there is no cause for concern. However, when the educator's perspective (which must necessarily take account of internal organizational survival issues) leads to specification of standards which relate to levels of internal institutional support, these may be irrelevant to the public purpose of accreditation. Indeed, the accreditation process, whether specialized, programmatic, or institutional, may be perverted to provide a dean, a department chairman, or a program director with more leverage on the parent institution for additional resources. Likewise, the external validation received through the accrediting process can legitimize a school or a program which, in the prevailing view of the internal academic community, is marginal. These concerns have, at best, an indirect relationship to the public or consumer purposes served by accreditation.

While most are in agreement with Dr. Kralewski's observation that an effective accreditation process should not be directive or prescriptive, once standards are adopted and increasingly tied to eligibility for extramural funding, the convergence on the standard model will surely follow. My overriding concern with accreditation in an emerging field of endeavor is the premature adoption of standards which precipitates a convergence on the current state of the art and which may also have the effect of discouraging new approaches or experimentation with other models.

Organizational Setting

Regarding the third issue of program location, I am not as sanguine as Dr. Austin that the issue of organizational locus has been laid to rest. On the contrary, I believe this issue should be continually debated, but not in terms of the old formulations which argued the merits of health-oriented versus management-oriented academic bases. Perhaps this formulation of the issue of location has subsided in the face of evidence that programs of excellence and mediocrity exist in both settings. I would suggest a reformulation of this topic of organizational base in terms of requirements or criteria applicable to any academic unit which seeks to develop a program. The first consideration is the comparability between the practice setting and the training or educational setting.

Bennis has predicted that we will witness the breakdown of our dominant organizational form, i.e., hierarchical bureaucracy, and the rise of newer social systems of organization better suited to contemporary demands. The contributing factors to this breakdown will be: "rapid and unexpected change; growth in size beyond what is necessary for the work being done . . . ; complexity of modern technology . . . ; a change in managerial values toward more humanistic democratic practices."[6] Thus the practice setting will require a manager with competencies to cope with this changing scene.

The university community often attempts to respond to these futuristic demands by producing the multidisciplinary scholars and professionals who have mastered two or more disciplines (as opposed to the interdisciplinary specialist). Campbell presents an alternative model— one of "collective competence." This alternative is presented to counter "the aspiration to produce modern day Leonardos who are competent in all of science." As I have already suggested, the major obstacle to Campbell's alternative of collective competence is the dominant organizational form of the university and the academic disciplines within its walls. This form and its organizational dynamics resist interdisciplinary initiatives in favor of departmental prerogatives.

The challenges for new approaches in the educational setting to match the demands in the practice setting are summarized by Bennis: "The new organizational forms will be adaptive, rapidly changing temporary systems, organized around problems to be solved . . . arranged on organic rather than mechanical models . . . where people will be evaluated, *not* in a rigid vertical hierarchy according to rank and status but flexibly according to competence."

If the educational setting (e.g., the locus of the program) is to bear any resemblance to the practice setting, then the following issues must be addressed:

Are the administrators of health services to be trained in survival and maintenance techniques for the dominant organizational forms, risking early obsolescence, or are they to be trained for the leadership styles required by the newer forms? Obviously, a mix is required, and the real issue is determining and rapidly adjusting that mix in a university setting more accustomed to a rigid than to a flexible curriculum.

A second set of issues involves the discrepancy between what the university teaches—the systems approach, organizational behavior, optimization, and cost containment—and the internal application of these principles to the design of instructional systems. The question here is whether the university setting provides appropriate role models and organizational models to reinforce the formal instruction.

The third issue is the positive transfer of training from the instructional setting to the practice setting. University faculties are fond of the claim that they teach principles which are applicable in a variety of settings; but knowing the principle and applying it require two different types of learning. Do university settings provide for the application of skills in a sufficient variety of settings to enhance or permit the positive transfer of training?

The fourth issue is set in the context of collaboration between the educational and practice settings. What are the mechanisms for this collaboration between the educator and the practitioner? What are the responsibilities and challenges for the university to collaborate with individual learners and their institutions in the design of the total process?

The fifth issue is one of determing the primacy of competencies expected from a graduate professional program. Perhaps some rethinking of these priorities is in order, given the role of the university and other continuing education enterprises. The current focus is clearly on partial, technical competence in a variety of techniques (including operations research, management science, and computer technology), with little or no emphasis on interpersonal skills or the underpinning of humanistic values prerequisite to the management of human factors in the labor-intensive industry.

I would suggest that all these are areas of inquiry which must be addressed by an organizational base which purports to educate or train administrators and managers of the health care enterprise. One may derive standards and criteria for quality programs from these issues and attempt to frame them in broad terms to deal more with general organizational characteristics than with specific inputs. An ideal instructional program would contain the following features to meet these challenges and resolve these issues:

The goal of the program is to produce interdisciplinary specialists with a core of interpersonal competence.

The environment should allow for three operating modes (service, research, and training) to accommodate the acquisition of basic principles and their application in the laboratory and in the real world.

The components of the instructional system should include the learner, his institution, and the training institution.

The resources available to the instructional system should include service, research, and training organizations, and rewards for collaboration and interchange of personnel and products.

The objectives of the program would be: to educate or train managers of health services programs, using a multidisciplinary faculty who relate to a unified leadership organization for their direction and rewards; to encourage faculty and students to identify interdisciplinary gaps and to develop specialized competence in filling those gaps; and to provide short- and long-term training experiences to fulfill the need for continuing professional development.

Systems maintenance activities should be provided to ensure feedback, redundancy, and systems correction. Redundancy is a requirement before faculty interchange across service, research, and training modes can be effected. Systems correction capability implies a leadership organization with authority and responsibility for the mix of resources and operating modes.

Without these characteristics the setting may be judged at least unreliable or at worst insufficient. Thus, in my view, the locus issue is still a real issue and must be assessed.

Jerry W. Miller, Ph.D.: Each profession has its own mystique. Some groups are more successful than others in maintaining that mystique and thereby claiming that it is in the social interest for them to maintain a great deal of autonomy. The mystique of a profession thickens when the topic becomes the quality of its education programs. A layman who tries to penetrate the mystique can be made to look very foolish, and sometimes with justification. Given other, too-obvious limitations, the situation today argues very forcefully against my taking that tack. Rather than commenting on John Kralewski's points, perhaps I can be most helpful by extending his comments. I do so as one who maintains continuing interest in the professions, their development, processes, and procedures, and their impact on education. Therefore, I want to comment on processes and procedures which have varied impact on the quality of education programs for health administration, some of which limit the autonomy of the profession, but not much. There are several kinds of quality control procedures which affect education for health care administration.

State regulation such as chartering or program registration. The impact of regulation of this kind is very broad and general, is virtually nonexistent in some states, and has little significance except for very minimal standards of quality. It provides protection only against bogus programs—degree-mill efforts.

Regional accreditation. This also is a very general type of quality control procedure, but it is a level above that provided by state government regulation. It says something about the adequacy of internal quality control procedures and decision-making processes within the institution. Its gross limitation is that it cannot provide an in-depth review of specific programs where closer scrutiny and third-party review are needed—to serve educational interests and to provide some protection of the public health, safety, and welfare.

Institutional quality control procedures. Institution-wide policies and procedures for faculty appointments, promotion and tenure, and curriculum approval exert some influence on the quality of programs in education for health administration. These procedures and policies have their roots in, and therefore are more germane to, the more established disciplines and professions. Consequently, such policies and procedures may not accommodate the uniqueness of a developing field. These intra-institutional considerations, if not inflexibly ˙ applied, are useful benchmarks of quality, though far from the last word. They at least warrant lip-service from the health administration faculty if the latter are to coexist with their colleagues in other disciplines.

I come now to procedures in which the profession can have the most influence.

The marketplace. Theoretically, the marketplace could be the only and final determinant of quality control. That, however, unreasonably assumes:

—An oversupply of graduates when there may be an undersupply.

—Recognition and reward of competency by decision makers in the marketplace.

—The nonexistence of an *old-boy network* which has a significant impact on employability, which provides excellent apprenticeship training opportunities for the graduate, and which therefore becomes a species of self-fulfilling prophecy.

—Nonintervening variables such as formal and informal postgraduate educational opportunities, and the lack of variety in individual motivation.

Nevertheless, the marketplace is a quality control factor, because in time it will eliminate opportunities for the hopelessly ill prepared and will therefore eliminate those educational programs that produce them.

Professional interaction and communication. Professional journals, conferences, and associations, because they channel and formalize intellectual activity addressing issues and problems, are obviously additional phenomena which influence the quality of education. Ideally, they involve practitioners, the academy, and related professions and disciplines.

Professional certificates, licensure, and regulation of health care delivery. In most professions, these are additional means for determining performance quality, and they obviously have some correlation with the quality of educational programs. Therefore, in ways that are not always readily identifiable, they affect educational programs.

Specialized accreditation. This process may be the most precise and the most promising for shaping the quality of education. At this point in the development of health administration and its educational programs, prudent attention to the accreditation process may be a good use of energy and resources, and may produce good results. The process of debating and setting standards and applying them to educational programs may be the best mechanism available for dissipating the mystique of education for health administration and for making more tangible the intangibles of quality. It is a process which forces attention on the specifics of the educational process and because it results in actions which directly affect programs and people, directs communication and thinking in tangible ways to the caliber of educational programs. Thus accreditation standards are, in most cases, statements as specific as can be made about the components needed for quality in educational programs; are usually the result of a consensus judgment of recognized experts in the field; are tested each time they are applied; and are applied by the recognized experts in the field, thereby facilitating communication and debate on the hard issues of achieving quality in health administration education.

Accreditation is a good method, but it is fraught with complexities that require a balancing act. It is being used not only to determine quality but also to explicate and give identity to an evolving field; it must somehow be used to determine quality without being too directive and to define quality without being too limiting. I'm not suggesting that we rely exclusively on accreditation. Rather, my perspective suggests that those of us who are

138

interested in the quality of education for health administration have a strong interest in making all of these processes contribute to the quality of education, but that we not permit any of them to obtain a stranglehold on the field or to exercise an undue influence. Pluralism and diversity have merits in every human endeavor, and especially in social and professional control.

None of these, obviously, is a fail-safe procedure. As far as I know, there are no fail-safe procedures where human endeavor is involved. They are nonetheless socially and educationally useful. Pluralism and diversity are especially important in a field where there is a lack of consensus among academicians and among practitioners, and where academicians and practitioners may be even more at variance. I perceive that this is the case in health administration.

Relax a bit. You will experience your future, and given social force you will probably have a large part in determining it, but you won't determine it exclusively.

Discussion

Joanne E. Finley, M.D. (presiding): Very quickly I'd like to make a comment that may stir up some discussion. In addition to my other responsibilities, I also administer a licensure program for a number of health disciplines, and also an institutional licensure program for nursing homes and hospitals, and I have become violently opposed to licensure as a measure of anything. In a large state program I have only one authority that I consider of any use to tell us whether we're protecting the public or not, and that is a clinical laboratory improvement bill which is based entirely on outcome measures of efficiency. So I have a very strong opinion in this area.

Time for general discussion was limited, and the discussion related to a single question about the methods used by the programs to select and guide students: "Some

139

of us are perhaps constrained by the idea that the GRE may be an excellent screening device, but there are other ways to look at students and to provide individuation of the curriculum," said the questioner. "I'd be interested to know what methods are being used to allow students not so much to be screened out as to be counseled and tracked. What kinds of methods are being used in the programs in some formal sense to identify student problems and to measure faculty performance?"

Responding, Dr. Kralewski said he was concerned about the trend toward screening examinations that attempt to qualify student competency. "I think there's a whole range of other attributes that we have to consider." A second concern, Dr. Kralewski said, is the method by which students select specific institutions and areas for study within the broad general field of health administration.

> I think the field has to play a much more active role in both these issues," he declared. "I think we can tell a lot more about the way students who have had some experience in the work setting will perform after they're through the graduate program. Second, I think there is a better opportunity for them to sort out the field and to decide where they want to be. Experience in the work setting would be a real advantage in sorting that out. We try to provide that in our program by providing the students with an opportunity to talk to administrators in various settings at the beginning of the year and to make some sort of selection for their field experience during the summer, so they may select a planning office, or a hospital, or a group practice, or whatever.

Dr. Kralewski acknowledged that the method is uncertain, and that there are many change-overs between the selection of field experience and actual choice of field upon graduation.

The discussion ended with a comment from a business school representative. "You'll all be interested to know that the business schools have solved this problem. You take 200 times your undergraduate average plus

140

your GRE score. If it equals 950 you're in and if it's less than that you're out, and I don't know what this debate is all about." A health administration program director had the last word: "We don't have access to that multi-dimensional dart board."

Notes

[1] John W. Gardner, *Excellence* (New York: Harper and Row, 1971), p. xvi.

[2] Fred F. Harcleroad and Frank G. Dickey, *Educational Auditing and Voluntary Institutional Accrediting* (Washington, D.C.: American Association for Higher Education, 1975), p. 2.

[3] Jerry W. Miller, "Accreditation: Voluntary versus Government," Remarks at the Federation of Associations of Schools of the Health Professions, December 13, 1972, Washington, D.C., p. 4.

[4] Ibid.

[5] Donald T. Campbell, "Ethnocentrism of Disciplines and the Fish Scale Model of Omniscience," in Sherif and Sherif, *Interdisciplinary Relationships in the Social Sciences* (Chicago: Aldine Publishing Company, 1969) pp. 329–348.

[6] W. G. Bennis, "Post-Bureaucratic Leadership," *Trans-Action*, July-August 1969, pp. 44–61.

IX

Health Administration
in the Context of
Financing Higher Education

Gary L. Filerman, Ph.D.: It is appropriate that a series of papers commissioned by the W. K. Kellogg Foundation to address the future of health administration education should include the subject of financing. The Foundation's contribution to the development of the health administration role in our society has been largely financial. Creating, demonstrating, stimulating, and even inveigling—all these strategies, and others—have been employed in what is one of the truly noteworthy accomplishments of an American foundation.

The Foundation's investments brought hospital administration graduate programs from isolated experiments to an established component of higher and professional education. The growth of the programs' capacity, quality, and impact coincided with, and substantially contributed to, a managerial revolution in Canadian and U. S. health care delivery. Despite all the management problems of the present, significant improvement in the public welfare can be attributed to knowledge, skills, and values contributed by men and women attracted to the field, and prepared for it, by programs developed with the support of the Foundation.

In the 20 years between the 1954 Kellogg Commission Report and the 1974 Report of the Commission on Education for Health Administration, the Foundation was joined, and eventually largely supplanted, as the financier of new programs, by the federal government and by the provinces. The Foundation's strategy shifted to an emphasis on faculty development, upgrading the practitioner, and developing the educational infrastructure. The federal government, at the very end of the period of expanded support for higher education, developed a parallel but less consequential thrust. The most significant trend during the 20 years has been toward financing graduate and undergraduate health administration education in the ways in which education for more established fields is supported. The Foundation, however, continues to be the primary source of support, and in many cases the creative spark, for innovation toward a more effective profession.

The objective of this paper is to identify the interfaces of the problems of financing health administration education and financing higher education. The intent is to delineate characteristics of education for this field which will influence its long-range support.

Programs in health administration are creatures of two worlds, health and higher education. Because the programs educate members of the health professions, there is a natural tendency to view them in terms of traits shared with the other health professions' educational programs and schools. In general, however, both the graduate and undergraduate programs have more in common with programs outside the health field than with programs of education for the other health professions. The extent of common ground differs, primarily in response to the programs' administrative settings and the degrees offered. Even those programs most integrated into professional schools which are relatively isolated from the greater university have been moving in an interdisciplinary direction—which increasingly exposes them to developments that affect higher education in general. Further, the tightness of resources in all higher education has tended to reduce the autonomy of the health sciences, with the result that schools of medicine, allied health, and public health are increasingly accountable to central administrations. Indeed, they increasingly look to the central administration for financial support. We are well into the period of adjustment dictated by changes in the pattern of government support and by inflation. Financing education for health administration, graduate and undergraduate, must be viewed in the context of the changing financial circumstances of the total university. The perspective must in fact be broader, taking into consideration multi-university systems and other external pressures for planning and regulation.

It is erroneous to look to a single source (the federal government) for the solution to the present financial problems of programs or for meeting the demands on the programs in the future. There are now universities which will not seek or accept certain federal grants or contracts because of an unwillingness to contend with the distortion of fiscal integrity which is involved. Others are concerned with distortions of institutional purpose, priorities, or values. Much of this response is a reaction to the now apparent effects of years of "going after" federal support.

If a university or its graduate-level commitment is financially shaky, a program which is richly supported from outside is a questionable investment, because the supporting academic structure may not be able to respond appropriately. This is not to say that existing programs in financially troubled institutions should not be supported; but program faculties must become knowledgeable about the issues in financing higher education nationally and within their provinces or states. Existing programs will have to respond positively to their institutions' efforts to grapple with the situation and must aggressively seek multiple kinds and sources of support. Institutions seeking to launch new programs should have to demonstrate that they are committed to sustaining quality programs in order to qualify for support from outside sources. If they do not, the result will be more inadequately supported and staffed programs. There are too many such programs now.

The shifts in federal policy which are having impact on the climate of higher education have a universal "bottom line" —less money, or no growth, which mean the same thing, coming on top of inflation. The changes go far beyond reductions in formula grants for health administration or allied health grants for undergraduate education. They include the precipitous drop in support for most kinds of fellowships and

144

traineeships that has hit every discipline, and most sharply just when health administration programs have been aggressively reaching out to other disciplines for collaboration. Other new developments include the decrease in the number of individuals receiving G. I. Bill funds and .plans to discontinue such benefits. There has been a sharp cutback in support for minority students, at the time when health administration is finally confronting the imbalances in participation in the field. Other examples abound in the United States —and in Canada—where the impetus for such change is at the provincial level.[1]

One result is new attention to the role of the states in financing higher education. The interest in state activity is partially due to federal emphasis on reversing the trend toward centralization in the national government, the best example of which is revenue sharing. It is also due to efforts by the higher education community to develop state support to replace federal funds. A third factor is specific federal legislation encouraging the states to establish planning agencies, the so-called "1202 Commissions."

In July, 1976, the Carnegie Foundation for the Advancement of Teaching published a landmark study, *The States and Higher Education*. The report concludes that "coordination, regulation, and consolidation of higher education have been increasing rapidly at the state level."[2] Among the findings are these:

—Every state has some mechanism covering the entire public higher education sector.
—There are 28 coordinating agencies for the public sector, 19 of which are regulatory.
—Every state except Wisconsin has some form of "planning, coordination, or regulation" covering private colleges and universities.[3]

It should be clear that the primary impetus in these developments is the allocation and use of money. Where participation is not mandatory, it may be encouraged as a *quid pro quo* for various forms of state aid.[4] There are obvious parallels with developments in health services delivery.

One of the most important aspects of state review and

145

planning is an emphasis on productivity, traditionally anathema to academicians. But state legislatures are looking at educational systems formerly characterized by rising enrollments and rising federal funds. Now they have former junior colleges which have become four-year community colleges, state teachers colleges which have been designated universities, and state universities which have been designated senior colleges and graduate centers. As institutional ambition has risen, so has the price. But some of the assumptions upon which such "upgrading" was based have been proven wrong. Legislators are therefore less amenable to underwriting expensive programs for nonresidents and are much more prone to question empty classrooms, four-day–week contracts, and small classes.[5]

All kinds of measuring devices have appeared by which graduate programs are, or will be, measured. They include the familiar faculty-student, credit hour–contract, hour-degrees-granted types of ratios. They also include production process equations which measure cost-benefit and cost-effectiveness.[6] State governments have established budget offices (some that cross departmental lines and some within education departments) which apply management evaluation and productivity measurements to produce independent information on which legislators base resource allocation decisions. Generally, but not always, the hard decisions are left to the individual institutions, once the state has mandated the ceilings. In an increasing number of cases the states are deciding the fate of individual existing programs, and in many, if not most, states there is control of new offerings, at least in the public sector.[7] New York and California have reviewed doctoral programs one-by-one. New York reviewed every program regardless of setting; California reviewed only those in the state system. New York recently studied every master's program in the state. In the last five years, AUPHA has supplied data for planning purposes to perhaps a dozen state agencies.

The Carnegie study makes it clear that private schools are not exempt. Private University A argues that the state should not expand neighboring State School B while A's facilities are underutilized. The state replies that it must overcome the tuition barrier at the private school, and student aid subsidies are tied to A's participation in planning.[8] For any institution, public or private, the productivity issue requires an answer to the simple question, "How do we get more for less?" Clark Kerr has stated that this decade will see higher education move toward quasi-public–utility status.[9] The health field can offer useful experience.

In this climate, health administration programs have obvious advantages and disadvantages. Concern for the quality of management in health services is apparent and increasing, and responsive efforts by universities to improve management will be attractive to federal and state legislators. If the current federal health manpower support proposals are enacted, the programs will have support which will encourage and enable them to focus on exactly those services that are most likely to attract state support. The disadvantage to the programs is that the need to respond to particular needs within the system, such as ambulatory care, long-term care, and home health services, dictates an increase in specialized faculty to serve segments of the student body. This will frequently subject the program faculties to hard scrutiny, because they will fall outside the tolerances of management and planning ratios. But it would be a serious error to avoid small ratios by lowering admissions criteria, by expanding enrollments inordinately, or by failing to develop expertise and service capacity in high-priority areas.

A clear statement of purposes and a strategy for development which commits a health administration program to fulfillment of the broadest objectives of the university will ensure the application of appropriate criteria. The National Board on Graduate Education concludes:

> Our greatest concern is the potential damage to graduate education that could occur if states succumb to political pressures or adopt simplistic evaluation methods that fail to assess differences in purpose and in quality among graduate programs. We strongly believe that excellence in scholarship, research, and graduate education, where it currently exists, should be maintained and enhanced, and that graduate programs with an ap-

147

plied, practitioner focus, serving the needs of new clientele groups with different interests from the traditional doctoral student, must also be provided. There is a clear and pressing need for greater and more explicit differentiation of function among graduate programs in the United States, with different evaluative criteria applied to programs with different purposes and missions; state policies will be critical to this outcome.[10]

Given the application of such criteria, a program with a capital *P* will be supportable in the most competitive of state systems or within the individual university—without sacrificing quality.

All universities reflect these developments in various ways. The life of the program faculty member is affected. Economic security is as great an issue as it ever has been in higher education. The spread of faculty unions demonstrates this concern. Friction between faculty and presidents is often the result of emerging financial constraints and accountability. Schools are being reorganized for greater management clarity, if not efficiency. Deans and faculty are being forced to develop priorities, which in effect means the loss of jobs for some of their colleagues. Institutional funds for supporting services, travel, and libraries are increasingly scarce, and in many cases the traditional alternative sources for support have been terminated. This process has been going on for five years and will continue until some fundamental restructuring of the institutions and expectations of educators has taken place.

A major characteristic of the restructuring should be noted as already evident. That is the emergence of the new clientele, including part-time students and those served by nontraditional delivery systems.[11] A recent American Council on Education report states, "The fact of central importance for postsecondary education today is that well over half of the student body (57.5 percent) participates on a part-time basis." It goes on to point out, "The fact that part-time students' participation is increasing at a rate three-and-a-half times greater than full-time enrollments lends impetus, even urgency, to this situation."[12] Health administration appears to be keeping up with this change. The Commission on

Education for Health Administration recommended specific attention to nontraditional education.[13] The Kellogg Foundation has responded by establishing a task force to explore the needs and potential of the field and to develop a program for implementation. The Accrediting Commission on Graduate Education for Hospital Administration is considering appropriate criteria for part-time study and has outlined an approach to the question of accreditation of nontraditional programs. These developments will facilitate timely adjustment on the campus by the health administration programs.

The interdisciplinary thrust of the programs may be blunted by the most straightforward effort to achieve accountability and to preserve resources at the departmental level. Accounting procedures which charge "home" programs for cross-registrants are becoming increasingly common. They encourage programs to keep students within the program and either to duplicate content available elsewhere or (most unfortunately) to omit it. It is to be hoped that programs will respond not by narrowing the curriculum, but by offering service courses of such quality and usefulness that they equalize, if not produce, revenue.

Faculty advancement is a serious problem on many campuses. Criteria for promotion and tenure are being applied more rigorously, and in some instances are being revised. Fewer tenured professors means less long-term commitment, more flexibility, and, in a way, more security for existing faculty. Programs in applied fields are tempted to hire only faculty members who can compete on the most traditional grounds; they specifically avoid candidates without doctoral degrees—including those with master's degrees and practical experience. The applied fields should be able to defend the need for the latter and to assure them that they have a fair chance for advancement. The defense rests on program quality, congruence with the aspirations of the institution, and most importantly, a demonstration of well-integrated and necessary program components.

This situation brings faculty development needs into sharp focus. The direct relationship between support for education in this field and the need for an effective faculty development program serving Canada and the United States cannot be overemphasized. There is an important role for AUPHA here, to provide opportunities and to overcome financial barriers.

In addition to developments in the economics of higher education, the role of states, and regulation, other issues in higher education significantly influence the climate of support for education for health services administration. These issues include: the place of the master's degree; the problem of achieving quality in professional education; the issue of degree designation; and the controversy over the need for more programs and graduates.

The problem of the place of the master's degree is that in some disciplines it is a way station on the road to a doctorate. This is relevant to health administration, because it is strongly practiced by the traditional disciplines in some institutions. It thus influences both the climate of support for programs terminating at the master's level and the value of the terminal master's degree for faculty status. The question most often approaches the intensity of an issue at those private schools where the public-service dimension of the terminal master's degree is least influential upon institutional charter.[14]

Some U.S. and Canadian programs in health administration provide professional education equal in quality to the best programs for any profession. By quality, I mean that the program encourages and demands the use of the students' full intellectual and (specifically) analytic potential in an environment that is both critical and supportive. It means that there are programs which allocate sufficient faculty time to students so that they can receive personal guidance, and that the faculty uses the time for that purpose. It has nothing to do with the number of students enrolled per se, nor with the number of full-time faculty. On the other hand, there are some programs, a minority, which are of a lower quality than the field should sustain. These are programs in which the faculty members demand little of themselves, let alone of their students, and where pseudoprofessionalism is substi-

150

tuted for the rigor required to prepare health administrators for real-world demands.

There seems to be a frequent but not inevitable conflict between quality and credentialism. The problem is most acute where professional programs are so captured by client agencies that the agencies dictate the standards—by dominating student selection as well as performance standards. This problem is inherent in the thrust of the recent Milbank Commission Report.[15] Programs which abnegate quality considerations in favor of credentialism may justify their position as assuring greater access to professional education or as public service. But awarding advanced degrees for work which is clearly not of graduate level, to individuals who cannot perform at the graduate level, is a disservice to the greater public which awards status to the credential. Such programs will not be supportable in the long run and will not enjoy the support of other faculty in competing for resources within the university. The academy will favor those whose work reflects positively on its standards.

It is too early to predict the effect of undergraduate health administration programs on their graduate-level counterparts. The common assumption is that the critical interface and adjustments will come in the marketplace for graduates. Another interface may be more critical and traumatic. Much of the teaching in the graduate programs is not at the graduate level. This is true of master's degrees in many fields, such as public health, business administration, and public administration. Some of the content is remedial; some of the information is elementary orientation to the profession. Other content is simply not covered in a rigorous manner. When the undergraduate movement finally develops a cohesive mission, it will be subjected to the same pressures for quality that exist at the graduate and professional level. This will generate a new proclivity for graduate education to stand for a distinct intellectual accomplishment.

Quality programs and effete programs are found in all kinds of settings. Some of the weakest programs in this field are in institutions of great status, and conversely, some of

151

the quality programs are in institutions with relatively little international stature. Interestingly, some of the weakest have enjoyed the most stable financing, and some quality programs have to scramble for support every year. But, by and large, the latter have received support, however soft. There are academically poor programs among the accredited, but there are few students in academically and professionally strong programs that are not accredited. Those academically weak programs which are accredited are as a result of their own commitment to peer review, under considerable pressure to improve.

The problem of financing education for health administration is exacerbated by the range of quality which the degree represents. That is one reason why an effective accreditation effort is essential to the long-range vitality of this profession and to the fulfillment of its obligations to the public.

The reasons education for health administration offers a variety of degrees are well known. They are historical, philosophical, and accidental. As a spokesman in the political arena, I have argued that the plethora of degrees granted in the field represents a diversity of educational approaches that is of direct benefit to the world of practice. In accreditation circles, I have described the diversity as symbolic of resistance to standardization and as an accreditation mechanism responsive to institutional prerogatives. The implications of this pattern are, however, more varied than such positions imply.

From the perspective of those who are in positions to provide support for health administration programs, the nature of the training represented by this plethora of degrees is unclear. Although physicians and veterinarians work in many settings, play many roles, and are in fact the product of a variety of educational approaches, the single label within each profession communicates a sense of continuity and common ground among the approaches to training and, perhaps more importantly, indicates agreement as to what education content is needed. In a forthcoming book, Loebs and I argue that there is an accepted core common to all settings in health administration education and that the

152

philosophic arguments about different degrees (particularly M.P.H., M.B.A., and M.P.A.) operate at a different level.[16]

In practice, I take every opportunity to urge a common degree, the M.H.A. The most compelling reason is that it puts a role-specific label on a product, which is far more supportable in the long run than is the current array of academic credentials. At the outset, the individual program faces a variety of choices. The degree choice is most often dictated by administrative considerations specific to the setting and the moment. A broader and more long-range appraisal of the options might well conclude that the interests of the institutions in gaining solid support and the interests of the profession are best served by a single, specific, and common designation.

Assuming that public recognition of the importance of the health administration role is achieved, the question remains, "Do we need any more health administrators than will be produced with the present form or level of support?" The answer depends on one's definition of the field in relation to the master's degree. Without engaging in the numbers debate, suffice it to say that the lack of consensus weakens the case for support.

The narrow view of the field, namely that its central mission is either the education of the top management of large general hospitals or of public health departments and their functional specialties, reinforces the most conservative estimates of need, and therefore undermines the case for support when *need* means *number*. There are plenty of applicants for top management jobs in large general hospitals (over 100-beds), and the future role of traditional public health departments is unclear.

Programs focusing almost exclusively on the traditional roles are less supportable, because they do not also contribute to the improvement of public services at points at which the needs are most clear. These are the points of service at the periphery of an outward-looking delivery system. It is important to note, however, that this is not a plea for programs that produce a "Jack-of-all-trades and master of none." Only distinctive competence[17] of both the program and its

153

graduates will merit support. It is a plea for "Johnny-on-the-spot and master of one."

Professional education requires educational involvement with the profession. There are health administration programs which are academically excellent but professionally ineffective because they have inadequate professional involvement. Involved programs are ultimately more supportable, because they are perceived as responsive to what the public needs from the profession. Academic excellence and professional involvement are compatible. There are several outstanding examples. But some excellent programs are not involved, confining themselves to a narrower base of support.

There is an appropriate role for the public sector in supporting graduate programs in the United States and Canada. But from the perspective of relative contribution to public service, not every venture in teaching health administration has an equal claim on such support. In the long run, the main criterion for support will not be accreditation. It will be one criterion among several touching on elements of the scope of a program. Accreditation addresses only the function of educating entry-level practitioners and, as we have noted, academic excellence in a practice vacuum must be its own reward.

To maintain competance and to progress, a health profession must interdigitate closely with an academic infrastructure. In the absence of multiple ties between practice and education, each becomes stultified and conservative. The profession, in particular, assumes a stance protective of its role, knowledge, and status—which only encourages obsolescence. For these and other reasons, the profession and the public expect educational programs to be broadly involved in the day-to-day experience of the profession. This involvement requires a scope of activities which is broader than master's or bachelor's degree production. There is a strong rationale for public support of the activities which constitute such involvement, and of the critical mass of faculty which implements them.

A program in health administration requires access to expertise in relevant disciplines such as sociology, epidemiology, systems engineering, economics, and statistics. It requires internal capacity in such functional areas as hospital administration, health planning, and mental health administration, as well as in research methodology and continuing education. To respond to the delivery system, each program should offer depth in two or more functional areas. This gives the student the option to pursue individual interests and keeps the program focused on the interplay of forces in the system rather than on one isolated component. Functional depth provides faculty resources for elective courses, research, continuing education, consultation, and community policy development. In other words it is the substance and scope required for what I have called a capital *P* program. Functional specialization substantially increases the cost of the program and increases the student-faculty ratio. It also substantially expands potential sources of support and increases the program's competitiveness.

A graduate program with 25 graduates in each of two years requires a minimum true budget on the order of $200,000 to achieve functional specialization. A true budget is composed primarily of funds which are managed directly by the program as an administrative entity. The critical question is who controls the funds, and not whether they are "hard" or "soft." The budget includes library acquisition allotments but excludes "in-kind" credit for faculty time earned through cross-registration with other departments, preceptor time, and other contributions by individuals who are carried on other budgets. It includes direct overhead but excludes indirect overhead.

The public's interest is in the services which a full-scope program provides to the delivery system. More effective health services result. There is an active involvement of faculty and students in the experience of practice. Such involvement is best accomplished without responsibility for the operation of a specific agency or program, a practice which may result in entanglements with vested interests. There is substantial evidence in public administration, agriculture, and public health that this is not a hypothetical concern and is for several reasons inimical to the achievement of quality.[18]

155

The needs in the health services delivery system to which the full range of program activities and services is addressed are largely attributable to a single source. That source is federal initiative in the organization and financing of services. The "state of undermanagement" derives not so much from the programs—Medicare, Medicaid, PSRO, HMO, and health planning in the United States, and hospital and medical insurance in Canada—as from the consistent lack of attention to the system's limited capacity to manage, which characterizes all of these programs.[19]

The complexity of demands on health management has grown faster than the system's ability to attract, train, and pay for competent administrators. Hospital administrators may generally disagree with this assessment, for the managements of large hospitals have been the most successful in coping with the requirements of implementing the legislation. These institutions have expanded management capacity, particularly through the addition of specialists in finance, information systems, and quality assessment, and have spread the cost over a comparatively large base.

This is not the case for many personal health service delivery entities, many of which are pivotal in efforts to de-emphasize the role of the large hospitals. Thus the state of undermanagement is most evident in group practice, prepaid group practice, nursing homes, homes for the aged, emergency medical care systems, neighborhood health centers, community mental health centers, home health agencies, small hospitals, and mental hospitals. Thus, there is a lack of trained management in the majority of delivery organizations. The result is inadequate care and poor utilization of available resources and, most importantly, a lack of creative entrepreneurship focused on realizing the objectives of the legislation.

Federal and provincial support of centers for health administration education is therefore a necessity. This support must be substantial and lasting, and it must support the full range of activities already described. The argument for supporting health administration education is more compelling than that for any other health profession, because unless the management-capacity gap is closed, the professions cannot contribute optimally to the accomplishment of national health objectives.

It has been argued that such support should be concentrated in the schools of public health.[20] That would ensure the continuation of the status quo. It has been well demonstrated that effective administrators, innovative leaders, and shapers of public policy are produced in programs in a variety of settings. In fact, programs in other settings have been more successful in attracting what is traditionally labeled "hard money." More important, such programs have enjoyed greater access to the best management and policy education resources on the campus, and have shown a far greater propensity to use it. The argument, however, is not one-sided. There are programs in public health which are among the leaders in exploiting such resources for the benefit of the health sector. But they do not stand out as a group, nor do the universities in which they are based stand out as having the resources to offer. Federal policy should focus on the need for public service and not on the survival of a particular educational entity.

After several years of effort, AUPHA has identified a pattern of public support for health administration education which is compatible with a number of public policy objectives. This pattern is based on the need for a full scope of service and educational activities by the programs. It requires a critical mass of students—but without tieing support to numbers, as in capitation. Potential and quality are recognized regardless of setting, and core support from nonfederal sources is required.

Thus, several desirable features are introduced into the federal health manpower system. Some proven pitfalls are avoided; among these is total dependence on federal support. Another undesirable outcome, overproduction, is at least not encouraged. The bottom line is that an institution which cannot earmark $100,000 for basic support cannot qualify for federal support and will not be able to compete. That is a modest commitment for quality professional education.

In summary, several characteristics of education for health administration which complicate the climate of support should

157

be recognized. The long-range financial viability of quality professional education will be determined largely by the individual and collective responses of the programs to university and community expectations. The challenge is for the programs to develop those characteristics which lure support.

Comment

Brian Biles, M.D.: The good news is that the new health manpower legislation does recognize health administration education and provides support for it. The bad news, of course, is that there's no money. Dr. Austin referred to the politics of retrenchment or the politics of scarcity, and I think that's the situation that we've been in and are likely to remain in. We can identify four factors with respect to health administration education.

One factor is that Richard Nixon won the last two elections, which means that from the highest levels on down through the OMB and the Secretary's office the emphasis has been on not spending any money, and on not initiating any new programs. This has meant that even when the Congress has moved to retain the existing programs of the Kennedy-Johnson years, these programs have been vetoed. I think it's important to remember that four of the last five HEW appropriation bills have been vetoed. So the problems facing this health field, and many health fields, over the last eight years have stemmed from very basic political decisions made by society.

The second point is that over the last two or three years we have had a recession; the economic situation has not been good, and this has meant a decrease in federal revenues and an increase in demands for expenditures in such areas as unemployment. This has reduced the resources available for new initiatives.

The third major factor affecting all health programs has been the unbelievable increase in the price of the financing programs, so that once you take the federal budget and divide it into health, welfare, education, housing, and whatever—and in health care there's a $5 billion increase for Medicare and Medicaid alone—nobody is likely to say "Yes, you can take that $5 billion, and here's another $5 billion to do some of the other things you want!" What they say is, "My God! Forty-two percent of the entire increase in the domestic budget was for Medicare and Medicaid! You can't possibly expect any money for other health programs!" Without any money at all for new initiatives—grants or elective types of programs—the increase in the health care budget has just been unbelievable.

The fourth point is that there has really been no constituency, no advocate, for health administration education. Even among the people whom you might expect to be interested in this area, health administration education is fourth or fifth on their lists. And when you say there are just a few extra dollars, they'll tell you to put it into medical education, mostly, or they may suggest some of it for nursing education, maybe the Hill-Burton program, or schools of public health—right down the line. And when they come in and get a chance to ask for one thing, nobody says, "What we'd rather have than anything else is just a few more millions for health administration education."

If we then look at the legislation produced in this atmosphere, both the House and the Senate authorization legislation provide new support for health administration education. There are three requirements for participation in the program: the program must be accredited; the program must have at least 25 students; and the program must have at least $100,000 in nonfederal support. The problem here has been one of boundaries. Everyone can recognize a medical school when they see it. People know what a school of public health is. But when you've got schools of business and schools of social work coming in, there's a great fear of being ripped off. The feeling has been that with the limited amounts we have, why should we give any of that money to a school of business or a school of social work? How do we really know this is a health program? The feeling now is that these requirements for accreditation, enrollment, and support might ensure that the money goes to volume programs which will train people who will actually go into the health field. There's not much money involved: the two bills variously provide between $2 million and $4 million for each of the fiscal years through 1980.

That's where we are today. This is the legislation that is likely to be enacted this year, and of course, as you people well know, appropriations are likely to be somewhat less than authorizations. Recognition, yes, but very little money—certainly nothing approaching a major new initiative.

If we then look to prospects for the future, if a Republican administration is elected, I think the prospects for new initiatives are virtually nil. The administration is recommending that the total health manpower appropriation be reduced from $500 million to $325 million. There's simply no room in that sort of budget for any new initiatives. If there is a Democratic administration, I think there are two possibilities: one is for some small increases, and whether we're talking about $2 million, $4 million, $3 million, or $6 million, those are the kinds of decisions that are made within the administration at the bureaucratic level, and I think the kind of people that are brought in by any Democratic administration would be willing to support small increases. Beyond that, the question of a major initiative depends on the whole national health insurance situation. If there is a Democratic administration and a national health insurance proposal, part of that program will be a very large cost containment package, and I think that package will include health planning, certificate of need, prospective rate setting, and utilization review. I suspect that health statistics may well be included. There will be a whole series of features. The question will be, how can we assure ourselves that the $20 billion or $40 billion or $60 billion program isn't going to increase at 15 percent a year? The advocates are going to be able to point to features in the bill and say, "The reason we know that isn't going to happen is that we have these features, and some of these of course are going to cost some money."

I would think that the question for advocates of health administration education is, can the products of the health administration programs be sold politically as effective cost containment? If the answer to that is yes, then there is some opportunity for increases in support for these programs. If the attempt is not made, or if the attempt is not persuasive, then I think that the federal resources for these programs will not increase.

Alvin L. Morris, D.D.S., Ph.D.: Being the last speaker at a conference can hardly be regarded as unique since someone fills that role at every meeting. Being the last of 21 formal speakers at a meeting which has spanned 40 hours is, nonetheless, unique for me. Since I can't mount a serious argument that they saved the best for the last, at least some satisfaction can be derived from having the last word.

Those of you who have had the pleasure of listening to Dr. Filerman's presentation will have the opportunity of reading his remarks in a publication which will result from this conference. My immediate reaction, after careful reading of his paper, was a reinforcement of my very real respect for the breadth and depth of his understanding of the factors which have impact on the field of health administration and the educational processes which sustain it.

Following a discussion of the economics of education, Dr. Filerman's comments were grouped under the following headings: place of the master's degree; quality; recognition; and the issue of need. Included under these headings one can find almost a laundry list of significant issues which are influencing both practice and education in health administration. While not all issues bear directly on financing of education, they develop, in an economic context, a concept of needs and demands in the field. Taken collectively, the issues suggest to me that

161

the key challenges of the future are related to a perception of the needs in health administration and the educational response to supplying the demands which are developing. However, as one from outside the field of health administration, I am led by Dr. Filerman's paper to the opinion that before these challenges can or will be met, the field must solve its identity problem.

It appears that those who need and purchase the services of health administrators and those who practice and teach in the field are all asking the question, "What is health administration, and what should it be?" How does one develop and recognize quality in health administration education when it is not clear what one should be teaching? How can maturity, recognition, and internal support in the academic setting be achieved when it is uncertain whether health administration is an undergraduate or graduate discipline or both, and when 13 different degrees can be granted to graduates in the field? In the face of these questions, the development of a sound financial base to sustain and expand education in health administration is an exceedingly difficult task. Building on Dr. Filerman's perceptive description of the "trees" in health administration, I would like to step back and spend a few moments taking a "forest" view of financing education for health administration.

Those providing leadership in health administration have made impressive strides in establishing the field as one of the health professions. While the impetus for seeking membership in the health professions is easily understood, it must be recognized that with that membership there are certain accompanying liabilities. Health administration now shares the frustrations, difficulties, and challenges being experienced by the broad field of health education. I would like to cite a few of these challenges for your consideration.

During the years from 1950 to 1970, a public policy in health services evolved in the United States. There now exists general public agreement that access to health services is the right of every citizen, and a heightened

162

expectation exists on the part of the people and the government which represents them. One of the problems which health administration has is that there has been no parallel development in public policy in health sciences education. Millis has pointed out that the vacuum caused by the presence of a public policy in health services and its absence in the education of health professionals is at the very root of the health crisis in our nation.[21]

The people of the United States are now exhibiting a great willingness to invest public and private funds in insurance for health services. Since services must be provided by trained manpower, it appears rational to look upon funds committed to health manpower education as insurance purchased by the healthy to assure the availability of manpower to provide services when needed. Perhaps it will take yet another score of years for a public policy to evolve which will support such a concept. In the meantime, health administration educators will be viewed by many as another platoon of health educators attempting to abscond with enough public funds to take a free ride and to do their own thing.

Those in the field of health administration must not be lulled into believing that all that is required to justify financial support for their educational programs is to describe the exciting and important services which the public should be anxious to receive from their graduates. It must be recognized that your goals for the nation's health do not coincide with society's goals. The prerogative of deciding what the people should want, should have, and should purchase in health does not rest with the health professions. As Fuchs has pointed out, every day, in manifold ways, Americans demonstrate that they place a higher value on satisfying other wants—and that health is not their most important goal.[22] The solutions put forth by health administrators as optimal for society will be disregarded unless they can be reconciled with competing needs and divergent priorities. They certainly will not form the basis for financial support, regardless of the sincerity with which they are defended. In the past, it has been comforting to assume that the public automatically wants the best we have to offer. The fact is that today we may have more in common with the Cadillac salesman than we would like to admit. We may be touting a product that is bigger, flashier, higher priced, and more expensive to run than the public really wants.

I can well understand that many in the audience may wish to counter these comments by pointing out that the thrust of health administration is to decrease costs and increase efficiency in health care delivery through better management. It may, therefore, seem logical to assume that expansion of the health manpower base by producing more health administrators would be welcomed by all. That such reasoning may not be productive was suggested in a recent paper by Dr. Rashi Fein:

> Discussions of health manpower often elaborate on the creation of new kinds of personnel and offer evidence or theory regarding the usefulness of such personnel in rationalizing the use of labor in the health industry. We are all aware of the articles that have been written and of the new experiments and demonstrations that have been mounted to show that new types of health professionals can add significantly to the efficiency of the health care delivery system; can economize on total resource use; and can, in many situations, improve quality. Such demonstrations are extremely valuable. Unfortunately, on occasion, many of us exhibit a tendency to assume that if we can demonstrate and document the fact that something makes sense, this will lead to the implementation of the newly discovered, sensible arrangements. Perhaps we are influenced by our understanding of the general economy in which it is alleged that if one builds a better mousetrap, the world will beat a path to his or her door. The health care market, however, is not financed in a fashion that provides sufficient incentive for the rationalization of labor inputs. In this particular market, we cannot simply assume that creating supplies of particular kinds of health professionals will necessarily lead to the creation of demand and of jobs for them . . . even when such personnel increase efficiency.[23]

164

The positive and constructive point which I have attempted to make is that leaders in health administration must be realistic as they seek to build a foundation of support for their educational programs. Merely possessing a better and much-needed mousetrap does not assure the emergence of that support, regardless of how well the story is told.

One of the special challenges faced by those who plan for the future of health administration is the complexity of the planning process itself. There was a time when planning was basically an intra-university process. Today, however, planning for health education is on the agenda of state legislators, state bureaus of health resources, state councils of higher education, and HSAs. What must be sought are more effective and efficient mechanisms for relating to these agencies.

In spite of the challenges to which I have alluded, I remain most optimistic about the future of health administration. It is a field whose time has come. It is important, however, that sufficient restraint be exercised to avoid the development of unrealistic expectations. While a compelling argument can be made for marked expansion of the field, of greater importance at this time is the attention to quality. A commitment to quality will mandate attention to the identity problem mentioned earlier. And when the identity of a health administration professional is clearly established, the process by which needs are identified and demands are met will proceed on a more rational basis. Also, as the identity is established the prospects for financial support of educational programs will be markedly improved.

Discussion

Karl D. Bays (presiding): We have a commitment to conclude this meeting at noon, so we have only a few minutes for questions and discussion, but we certainly want to take advantage of that time.

The opening comment suggested that the most important thought expressed during the conference had been the challenge put by Dr. Biles: Can the products of health administration education be sold as managers of cost containment? Cost containment is much more than just financial management and comprehends such concepts as quality, utilization review, certification of need, and other aspects of planning. "The more we train for financial management, the wider the gap is going to be between our products and the field," said a program director, "and I think we'd better look at that right now."

Following this comment, Mr. Bays asked Dr. Biles whether in his opinion the Senate subcommittee in its deliberations had given sufficient attention to issues of quality, as well as cost containment. "I agree with Dr. Morris," said Dr. Biles.

> We've got a Cadillac health care system, and I think that in the subcommittee the problem is not that the committee has been too little concerned with quality, but too much concerned. We can talk about the fact that the system is uneven, the technology issues, and everybody doing whatever they want to do, but if you look at the three basic problems—cost escalation, availability and accessibility, and quality—the political situation right now, the political problem now, is cost. The concern here and there may be that we might do more about availability and quality, but the real political problem, the basis on which you can get legislation enacted, the basis on which you can increase appropriations, is cost containment right now.

It was again suggested that we often lose sight of the fact that cost containment means control of utilization, not just price, and Dr. Biles agreed. He was reminded that one of the speakers had referred to "the regulators and the regulated," and he added:

> I think you've got to do a good job on both sides of that line. But the question with respect to health administration education remains: Can you persuade the politicians —federal, state, and local—that the products of these programs will do a significantly better job, will contribute to

the success of the health care system on both the regulator side and the regulated side, better than we would do if we just continued to hire people catch-as-catch-can from the M.B.A. programs? Do we really need training programs? Or do we in fact just need health programs? If we have programs, then people to administer them will come from somewhere. That's the key question, and I personally don't feel that it's been satisfactorily resolved by this discussion, and certainly not by the Commission Report.

Dr. Biles' comments raised a question of definition: If you become too discrete in your discipline or in your training and you think you're producing experts in cost containment who have been taught only financial management and efficiency or productivity and do not really understand all the tools and concepts of planning, then you're still not training people in cost containment.

"There's a political bottom line to this discussion," Dr. Filerman responded.

When I go padding through the halls of the Rayburn Building I feel a little bit like a pencil salesman—and that's usually the way I'm greeted, as a matter of fact. Because as Dr. Biles pointed out, health administration education is not on anybody's list. I'm all alone. There's no support—we don't have support of any significant variety from the field, from the AHA, or from any practitioner organization. In fact, in informal conversation last night it was pointed out that the obvious reaction from the field is that if they write a letter to their Congressmen asking for more support for health administration education, there will only be more competition for their jobs. What they ought to be doing instead is getting up there with me and pointing out what their contribution to these issues is. They're not doing that.

A final comment suggested that the conference had been struggling with the problem of identification for health administration that had been covered in the report of the Commission on Education for Health Administration, but had not dealt with the recommendation of the Milbank report that there should be education at the postprofessional level, directed to training certain postprofessionals not as administrators but as executives, policy makers, and planners. The next conference, it was suggested, might have to deal with further questions of identification, roles and responsibilities in financial management, cost containment, and quality issues for those executives in policy-making positions.

Notes

[1] Allan M. Cartter, "The Future Financing of Postsecondary Education," in *Education and the State*, ed. John F. Hughes (Washington, D.C.: American Council on Education, 1975), p. 52.

[2] Carnegie Foundation for the Advancement of Teaching, *The States and Higher Education*, (San Francisco: Jossey-Bass, Inc., 1976), p. 85.

[3] Ibid., p. 85.

[4] James A. Perkins, "Coordinating Federal, State and Institutional Decisions," in *Education and the State*, op. cit., pp. 188–189.

[5] William Toombs, *Productivity: Burden of Success*, ERIC/Higher Education Report No. 2 (Washington, D.C.: American Association for Higher Education, 1973).

[6] Philip H. Coombs and Jacques Hallak, *Managing Educational Costs* (New York: Oxford University Press, 1972), p. 82.

[7] Carnegie Foundation for the Advancement of Teaching, op. cit., p. 51.

[8] Allan M. Cartter, op. cit., p. 57.

[9] Kenneth Mortimer, *Accountability in Higher Education*, ERIC Report No. 1 (Washington, D.C.: American Association for Higher Education, 1972).

[10] National Board on Graduate Education, *Outlook and Opportunities for Graduate Education* (Final Report, No. 6) (Washington, D.C.: National Board on Graduate Education, December 1975), p. 20.

[11] Allan M. Cartter, op. cit., pp. 66–67.

[12] Committee on the Financing of Higher Education for Adult Students, *Financing Part-Time Students*, (Washington, D.C.: American Council on Education, 1974), p. 47.

[13] *Education for Health Administration*, Vol. I (Ann Arbor: Health Administration Press, 1975), p. 7.

[14] Bernard Berelson, *Graduate Education in the United States* (New York: McGraw-Hill Book Company, 1960), pp. 187–188.

[15] Milbank Memorial Fund Commission, *Higher Education for Public Health* (New York: Prodist, 1976), pp. 127–129.

[16] Gary L. Filerman and Stephen F. Loebs, "Education for Health Administration," in *Review of Allied Health Education II*, ed. Joseph Hamburg (Lexington: University of Kentucky Press, 1976) (in press).

[17] The notion of distinctive competence in the graduates of a program is adopted from Philip Selznick's concept that the character of an organization lies in its distinctive competence or lack thereof. See Philip Selznick, *Leadership in Administration* (Evanston: Row Peterson and Company, 1957) pp. 42–56.

[18] Milbank Memorial Fund Commission, op. cit., p. 132.

[19] U. S. Senate Committee on Labor and Public Welfare, *Health Professions Educational Assistance Act of 1976*, Report No. 94–887 (Washington, D.C.: U. S. Senate, 1976), p. 230.

[20] Milbank Memorial Fund Commission, op. cit., pp. 162–171.

[21] J. S. Millis, *A Rational Policy for Medical Education and Its Financing* (New York: The National Fund for Medical Education, 1971), p. 6.

[22] V. R. Fuchs, *Who Shall Live: Health Economics and Social Choice* (New York: Basic Books, 1974), p. 4.

[23] Rashi Fein, "Health Manpower: Some Economic Considerations," presented at the *Symposium on Health Sciences Education in the 21st Century*, sponsored by the University of California, Newport Beach, California, June 3, 1976.

BIBLIOGRAPHY

(Dr. Filerman)

AUPHA. *Faculty Salary Survey*. Washington, D.C.: Association of University Programs in Health Administration, 1976.

Bowen, William G. *The Economics of the Major Universities*. Berkeley: Carnegie Commission on Higher Education, 1968.

Carnegie Commission on Higher Education. *Quality and Equality: Revised. Recommendations: New Levels of Federal Responsibility for Higher Education*. New York: McGraw-Hill Book Co., 1970.

Fein, Rashi and Weber, Gerald J. *Financing Medical Education*. New York: McGraw-Hill Book Co., 1971.

Filerman, Gary L. "Issues in Program Development," *Undergraduate Education for Health Services Administration*. Washington, D.C.: Association of University Programs in Health Administration, 1975, pp. 27–34.

Honey, John C. and Hartle, Terry W. *Federal-State-Institutional Relations in Post-secondary Education*. Syracuse, New York: Syracuse University Research Corporation, 1975.

Mayhew, Lewis B. *Reform in Graduate Education*. Atlanta: Southern Regional Education Board, 1972.

Mayville, William V. *A Matter of Degree: the Setting for Contemporary Master's Programs*. ERIC Report No. 9, 1972. Washington, D.C.: American Association for Higher Education, 1973.

Panel on Alternative Approaches to Graduate Education. *Scholarship for Society*. Princeton: Educational Testing Service, 1973.

Powel, John R., Jr. and Lamson, Robert D. *Elements Related to the Determination of Costs and Benefits of Graduate Education*. Washington, D.C.: Council of Graduate Schools, 1972.

Schein, Edgar H. *Professional Education: Some New Directions*. New York: McGraw-Hill Book Company, 1972.

Snell, John L. "The Master's Degree." In *Graduate Education Today*, ed. Everett Walters. Washington, D.C.: American Council on Education, 1965, pp. 74–102.

X

Concluding Remarks

Robert A. DeVries: To close this two-day conference allow me, on behalf of the Kellogg Foundation, to thank each of you for your commitment of time, energy, and intellect and especially to express appreciation to the co-chairmen, Nathan Stark and Karl Yordy, to Gary Filerman for encouragement and ideas, and to George Bugbee for his extraordinary effort and genius in the construction and operation of the conference. For many of us, these have been rewarding hours as we have explored ways and means to improve health administration education and practice. Surely last night's all-star cast gave many of us a "leg up" on the subject.

I want you to know that the W. K. Kellogg Foundation intends to continue its substantial and long-standing interest in health care administration education programming. We believe much remains to be done to upgrade both the management and governance of health care organizations, and several of us have set about in a deliberate, active fashion to encourage progressive, experimental, nontraditional—yet practical and highly visible endeavors in this field. Immediately following the Report of the Commission on Education for Health Administration, our Foundation set in motion the implementation of selected recommendations such as the establishment of the two North American Task Forces on Centers for Advanced Study and Nontraditional Education and Lifelong Learning, which serve as bridges in implementing the data-gathering and interviewing activities of the Commission. Further, the Foundation has in the past two years proceeded with at least six awards totaling more than $2 million; each of which addresses one or more of the Commission's recommendations. These grants are to:

171

The University of Chicago Graduate School of Business for the development of a master's degree program for health executives who are not formally prepared but who wish to pursue part-time graduate education while continuing full-time health administration employment. This Health Executives Program is designed to meet the special needs of working executives who show particular competence and promise as managers. It operates off-campus in downtown Chicago.

The University of California, Berkeley, in behalf of an informal association of four faculties of accredited programs in health administration in the western United States (UC-Berkeley, UCLA, the University of Colorado, and the University of Washington), and in concert with the Association of Western Hospitals, for development of a work program for implementing the Commission's recommendations, especially those on continuing education. This western consortium is chaired by Dr. David Starkweather.

Northwestern University School of Management to establish a part-time master's degree program in health services administration for employed middle managers and chief executives in health institutions and organizations.

Hospital Financial Management Educational Foundation (Chicago), in conjunction with Tulane University, Ohio State University, the University of South Carolina, and the University of Colorado for a national, comprehensive hospital financial management educational program involving both graduate academic credit and HFMA certification, based on a national core curriculum and with the potential of leading to an external degree.

Center for Research in Ambulatory Health Care Administration of the Medical Group Management Association (Denver), for the development of a national continuing education program for ambulatory care and group practice administrators, the provision of pilot residency experiences for health administration students in ambulatory care settings, and for the production of teach-

172

ing materials for the in-service training of middle-level ambulatory care supervisory personnel.

Trinity University (San Antonio, Texas), for the establishment of a regional center to provide programs of lifelong learning and nontraditional education on an individualized basis for long-term care, mental health, and hospital administrators.

I hope these recent Foundation awards will give you some idea of our continued active interest and clear commitment to health care management education. I sincerely hope this conference has stirred your thoughts and energies for effecting changes and for the implementation of additional Commission recommendations; we are expecting great things—creative strategies and new initiatives—from you, and we promise to look with great care at the directions suggested for advancing the field and promoting the public good. Certainly the Kellogg Foundation stands ready to do its part, along with many other agencies, associations, professional societies and state, provincial, and federal governments in this important mission.

Thank you again for coming.

XI

Feedback

In the weeks following the conference the sponsors received a number of letters from those who had attended. One program director described the conference as "one of the most intellectually stimulating that I have attended in years," and an educator from outside the health field characterized it as "an important event in moving health administration further in the direction of professionalism." Another program director thought "The meeting went well except for the role of apologist taken by several practitioners."

Some of the comments went beyond an assessment of what was said, to its implications—what Dr. Mawby had referred to as *so what?* An observer from outside the health field found it refreshing "that academicians and practitioners are not complacent about the profession, but are seeking to improve it and to make it one of the truly learned professions. Continued assessment of the training of health administrators is critical if those administrators are to be commensurate in ability with the complexity of the challenges in the health care field." A practitioner stated that he had gained "a much better understanding of the issues relating to health administration education. Because of this sensitivity, I can be more supportive of some of the efforts and activities that will make these educational programs more effective and efficient."

As always, there were criticisms. One view was that the general discussions were "good in spots but very unproductive in others"—a common failing of general discussions. Another comment was that there were too few practitioners present and that it would have been helpful to have more "employers of the product." The most critical and comprehensive and, in many ways the most thoughtful, of all the comments came from a member of the emerging health administration specialty—health planning. Samuel S. Long, Executive Director of the Health Planning Association of Northwest Ohio, found the conference most interesting with respect to his concern for the performance of Health Systems Agencies and the credentialing of health planning staffs. Mr. Long's letter continued:

Graduate schools of health and hospital administration are generally not in close communication with me or my colleagues. However, I begin to sense that undergraduate schools in health administration are making some attempts to communicate regularly. This may be due to their local nature, but it is a movement that graduate educators should consider. The graduate schools rarely ask advice and when they do, through conferences or advisory committees, my colleagues and I see too little evidence that the advice is received, understood, or acted upon. There is a need for a bridge between graduate educator and practitioner, and the bridge must be built from both sides. Some experience with the process and product of such building would be welcome. The graduate program might assign a staff person to work with, and be responsible for, liaison with the Health Systems Agencies in the area of interest to the program. Thus the university could offer the services of a staff member to meet periodically with HSA directors. Most states are organized. In Ohio, one person could cover the ten HSAs with one meeting.

HSAs should respond by offering their assistance as a teaching resource to the graduate and undergraduate educational process. An HSA is, and can be, a valuable teaching resource both as a community laboratory and as a field center for students in training and in residency.

Educational institutions must face up to some overwhelming internal problems which affect their credibility with planners. They have in too few instances developed a capacity for inter-institutional or intra-institutional cooperation. My prediction is that undergraduate programs will recognize this and will precede graduate programs in intra- and inter-institutional coordination in their teaching programs.

In short, the bridge won't work without total commitment

to the process; otherwise the credibility of the programs is questionable. I believe this also pertains to hospital administration. The instances of hospital cooperation are growing and should be encouraged. In fact, one could argue that educational institutions have contributed mightily to division and conflict and only meagerly to cooperation and coordination; students are well aware of the unbridled competition and uncooperativeness of prima donnas on the faculties of many of our institutions.

The cure is not condemnation but a system of positive incentives that would contribute to change toward new objectives of maintaining autonomy but with cooperation, coordination, and joint effort. Competition can be maintained and improved as competitive efforts to reach these goals are encouraged.

Universities and graduate programs must provide leadership for health administration, health planning, and health education. HSAs need a place to look to for intellectual direction. That intellectual direction should be developed in cooperation with HSAs. We know what we need to some extent, and to some extent we have to be taught. These matters could be aided by building the bridge. Forced feeding, by seeking HEW grants for research and then descending on the field with great dissertations, doesn't work well. Fruitful areas of research and analysis can be worked out to meet the needs of the universities, the students, and the HSAs, but only if they are in communication with each other.

I view health administration and health planning as not only compatible but almost synonymous. Some of our best planners are from schools of hospital and health administration and medical care administration. Planners must have the ability to analyze, think, and communicate, and to develop initiatives— all of which are essential to successful administration. We have a great deal to communicate.

Finally, continuing graduate education is essential to the relationship between education and practice. Here again, educator credibility and the bridge are essential for success. There is no greater need in HSAs today than for the continuing education of staff and volunteers. Educational institutions should provide the leadership and organizational base for this, in cooperation with one another and with HSAs. Educational needs can be defined and assigned priorities cooperatively if both groups are willing to work together.

XII

Participants

Charles J. Austin, Ph.D.*
Dean of Graduate Studies
Trinity University
San Antonio, Texas 78284

Karl D. Bays**
Chairman of the Board
American Hospital Supply
   Corporation
Evanston, Illinois 60201

Brian Biles, M.D.*
Professional Staff Member
Senate Health Subcommittee
U.S. Senate
4228 Dirksen Building
Washington, D.C. 20510

Calvin Bland
Program Officer
The Robert Wood Johnson
   Foundation
The Forrestal Center
P.O. Box 2316
Princeton, New Jersey 08540

H. Robert Cathcart*
President
Pennsylvania Hospital
Eighth and Spruce Streets
Philadelphia, Pennsylvania 19107

Harold Cohen, Ph.D.
Director
Maryland Health Facilities
   Cost Review Commission
201 West Preston Street
Baltimore, Maryland 21201

Harold J. Cohen*
Chairman
Administration of Health
   Services Program
School of Allied Health
   Professions
Ithaca College
Ithaca, New York 14850

Robert F. Corcoran
Associate Director
Post Secondary Education
   Department
Education Commission of the
   States
Suite 300, 1860 Lincoln Street
Denver, Colorado 80203

Robert M. Cunningham, Jr.
2126 North Dayton Street
Chicago, Illinois 60614

* Speaker or discussant
** Presiding

177

James P. Dixon, M.D.*
Consultant
Union for Experimenting
    Colleges and Universities
930 Corry Street
Yellow Springs, Ohio 45387

Charles C. Edwards, M.D.**
Senior Vice President for
    Research and Scientific Affairs
Becton, Dickinson and Company
Rutherford, New Jersey 07070

E. Frank Ellis, M.D.
Regional Health Administrator
Public Health Services
U.S. Department of Health,
    Education, and Welfare
300 South Wacker Drive
Chicago, Illinois 60606

Harold L. Enarson, Ph.D.*
President
Ohio State University
Columbus, Ohio 43210

Howard S. Ennes
Vice President for Health
    Affairs
The Equitable Life Assurance
    Society of the United States
1285 Avenue of the Americas
New York, New York 10019

Saul Feldman, D.P.A.
Director
Office of Mental Health
    Education and Staff
    Development
National Institute of Mental
    Health
Rockville, Maryland 20852

Gary L. Filerman, Ph.D.*
President
Association of University Pro
    grams in Health Administration
Suite 420, One Dupont Circle
Washington, D.C. 20036

Joanne E. Finley, M.D.**
New Jersey State Commissioner
    of Health
New Jersey State Department
    of Health
P.O. Box 1540
Trenton, New Jersey 08625

John R. Griffith, M.B.A.
Director
Program and Bureau of
    Hospital Administration
School of Public Health
University of Michigan
Ann Arbor, Michigan 48109

Jeannette V. Haase, Ph.D.
Director
Programs in Health Care
Radcliffe Institute
77 Brattle Street
Cambridge, Massachusetts 02138

James G. Haughton, M.D.**
Executive Director
Health and Hospitals Governing
    Commission of Cook County
1900 West Polk Street
Chicago, Illinois 60612

Lawrence A. Hill*
Executive Director
New England Medical Center
    Hospital
171 Harrison Avenue
Boston, Massachusetts 02111

178

George A. Huber, J.D.
Lecturer and Legal Counsel
Department of Health Services
  Administration
Graduate School of Public
  Health
University of Pittsburgh
Pittsburgh, Pennsylvania 15261

B. Jon Jaeger, Ph.D.
Chairman
Department of Health
  Administration
Duke University
Durham, North Carolina 27710

Herbert Klarman, Ph.D.
School of Public Health
Johns Hopkins University
Baltimore, Maryland 21205

Barbara K. Knudson, Ph.D.**
Dean
University College
University of Minnesota
Minneapolis, Minnesota 55455

John E. Kralewski, Ph.D.*
Director
Program in Health Administration
Department of Preventive
  Medicine
School of Medicine
University of Colorado
  Medical Center
Denver, Colorado 80220

Samuel S. Long, M.P.H.
Executive Director
Health Planning Association of
  Northwest Ohio
225 Allen Street
Maumee, Ohio 43537

Gordon K. MacLeod, M.D.
Chairman
Department of Health Services
  Administration
Graduate School of Public
  Health
University of Pittsburgh
Pittsburgh, Pennsylvania 15261

William H. McBeath, M.D.**
Executive Director
American Public Health
  Association
1015 18th Street, N.W.
Washington, D.C. 20036

Thomas McCarthy, Ph.D.
Assistant Administrator
Health System Liaison
Health Resources Administration
U.S. Department of Health,
  Education, and Welfare
Rockville, Maryland 20852

Carl A. Meilicke, Ph.D.
Department of Sociology
University of Alberta
Edmonton, Alberta
Canada

Derril D. Meyer
Vice President
King's Garden Senior Citizens'
  Community
19303 Fremont Avenue North
Seattle, Washington 98133

Jerry W. Miller, Ph.D.*
Director
Office of Educational Credit
American Council on Education
Suite 800, One Dupont Circle
Washington, D.C. 20036

179

Frank Moore, Ph.D.*
Associate Dean
School of Public Health and
  Tropical Medicine
Tulane University
New Orleans, Louisiana 70112

Alvin L. Morris, D.D.S., Ph.D.*
Executive Director
Association for Academic
  Health Centers
1625 Massachusetts Avenue, N.W.
Washington, D.C. 20036

Beverlee Myers, M.P.H.
Department of Medical Care
  Organization
School of Public Health
University of Michigan
Ann Arbor, Michigan 48109

Louis A. Orsini
Vice President and Director
Health Insurance Association
  of America
919 Third Avenue
New York, New York 10022

John M. Phin, M.D.
Executive Director
Canadian College of Health
  Service Executives
25 Imperial Street
Toronto, Ontario M5P 1B9
Canada

Haynes Rice
Assistant Administrator for
  Special Projects
Howard University Hospital
2041 Georgia Avenue, N.W.
Washington, D.C. 20060

William C. Richardson, Ph.D.*
Chairman
Department of Health Services
School of Public Health and
  Community Medicine
University of Washington
Seattle, Washington 98195

Frederick C. Robbins, M.D.
Dean
School of Medicine
Case Western Reserve University
Cleveland, Ohio 44106

Hugh Rohrer, M.D.
Director of Health
Peoria County Health
  Department
2116 N. Sheridan Road
Peoria, Illinois 61604

William R. Roy, M.D., J.D.*
Director of Medical Education
  and Professional Services
St. Francis Hospital
1700 West 7th Street
Topeka, Kansas 66606

Cecil G. Sheps, M.D.
General Director
Beth Israel Medical Center
10 Nathan D. Perlman Pl.
New York, New York 10003

Robert D. Sparks, M.D.
Program Director
W. K. Kellogg Foundation
400 North Avenue
Battle Creek, Michigan 49016

Nathan J. Stark, J.D.**
Vice Chancellor
Schools of Health Professions
University of Pittsburgh
Pittsburgh, Pennsylvania 15261

David B. Starkweather, Dr. P.H.
Chairman
Graduate Curriculum in
  Hospital Administration
School of Public Health
University of California,
  Berkeley
Berkeley, California 94720

Michael J. Stotts
265 River Road
Granview, New York 10960

Richard J. Stull
Executive Vice President
American College of Hospital
  Administrators
840 North Lake Shore Drive
Chicago, Illinois 60611

John D. Thompson*
Chief
Division of Health Services
  Administration
Department of Epidemiology
  and Public Health
School of Medicine
Yale University
New Haven, Connecticut 06510

Peter B. Vaill, D.B.A.*
Dean
School of Government and
  Business Administration
George Washington University
Washington, D.C. 20052

George R. Wren, Ph.D.
Director
Institute of Health
  Administration
School of Business
  Administration
Georgia State University
Atlanta, Georgia 30303

J. Albin Yokie*
Executive Vice President
American College of Nursing
  Home Administrators
4650 East-West Highway
Washington, D.C. 20014

Karl D. Yordy*
Senior Program Officer
Institute of Medicine
National Academy of Sciences
2101 Constitution Avenue, N.W.
Washington, D.C. 20418

**For the W. K. Kellogg
Foundation:**

Russell Mawby, Ph.D.
President

Andrew Pattullo
Vice President

Robert A. DeVries
Program Director

For the Conference:

George Bugbee
Coordinator
Professor Emeritus
University of Chicago

Lois Alsip
Administrative Assistant
421 West Grant Place
Chicago, Illinois 60614

181